THE COURTSHIP OF
TWO DOCTORS

THE COURTSHIP OF
TWO DOCTORS

A 1930s Love Story of Letters, Hope & Healing

MARTHA HOLOUBEK FITZGERALD

Editor

Based on the 1937–1939 correspondence of
Alice Baker M.D. and Joe Holoubek M.D.

Little Dove Press
Shreveport, Louisiana

LITTLE DOVE
PRESS

Copyright © 2012 by Martha H. Fitzgerald
Little Dove Press
3902 George Road, Shreveport LA 71107
318 429-6524
www.littledovepress.com

First Edition

Printed in the United States of America
Library of Congress Control Number: 2012936187

Publisher's Cataloging-In-Publication
The courtship of two doctors : a 1930s love story of letters, hope & healing / Martha Holoubek Fitzgerald, editor. -- 1st ed. -- Shreveport, La. : Little Dove Press, c2012.
p. ; cm.
ISBN: 978-0-9757366-3-8 (cloth) ; 978-0-9753766-4-5 (pbk.) ; 978-0-9753766-5-2 (ebk.)
"Based on the 1937-1939 correspondence of Alice Baker M.D. and Joe Holoubek M.D."
Includes bibliographical references.
Summary: In 1937 senior medical students from New Orleans, Louisiana, and Omaha, Nebraska, met at the Mayo Clinic and began a two-year correspondence. Their courtship letters shed light on early 20th century society, hospitals, and health care.
1. Holoubek, Alice Baker. 2. Holoubek, Joe Edward, 1915-2007. 3. Medical students--United States--Correspondence. 4. Interns (Medicine)--United States--Correspondence. 5. Physicians--United States--Biography. 6. Women physicians--United States--Biography. 7. Medical education--United States--History--1933-1945. 8. [Education, Medical--history. 9. Education, Medical--personal narratives. 10. Physicians, Women. 11. Women in Medicine--history.] I. Fitzgerald, Martha Holoubek. II. Holoubek, Alice Baker. III. Holoubek, Joe Edward, 1915–2007. IV. Title.
R154.H65 F58 2012   2012936187
610.92/273--dc23   1208

Adapted from "The Holoubek-Baker Letters: An Annotated Collection," Volumes I and II, by Martha H. Fitzgerald, editor, a research compilation. Copyright © 2008 Martha H. Fitzgerald and the Holoubek Family LLC. Family photographs and excerpts from unpublished diaries and memoirs of Joe E. Holoubek M.D., covering the years 1935–2007, used by permission of his heirs. All rights reserved. Used by permission. "Harbor Lights." Words and music by Jimmy Kennedy and Wilhelm Grosz . Copyright © 1937 (renewed) Peter Maurice Music Co., Ltd. All rights in the U.S. and Canada administered by Chappell & Co. All rights reserved. Used by permission.

Cover design and production supervision: Dunn+Associates, dunn-design.com
Author photo: Neil Johnson, njphoto.com
Interior design: Dorie McClelland, springbookdesign.com
Book consultant: Ellen Reid, indiebookexpert.com

In loving memory of my parents,
who taught their children
the meaning of forever love,
and with humble thanks to my husband,
whose ever-inquisitive mind
and tender heart continue to inspire me

CONTENTS

PREFACE
page ix

MEDICAL TRAINING
page xv

PROLOGUE
Rochester, Minnesota, 1937
page 1

ONE

SENIOR YEAR
Nebraska & Louisiana

'I have never met a girl like you'
August–September 1937
page 23

'I had better quit philosophizing'
October–December 1937
page 31

'Your voice sounded so nice'
January–June 1938
page 61

'One week was not enough'
June 1938
page 129

TWO

INTERNSHIP
Nebraska & Louisiana

'About Rochester . . .'
June–September 1938
page 145

'How I hate to write this'
September–December 1938
page 197

'Darling, please don't worry'
January–March 1939
page 267

'We can lick the whole world together'
April–June 1939
page 313

EPILOGUE
Alexandria, New Orleans & Shreveport
page 365

APPENDIX
Timeline
page 377

Family and Friends
page 378

Medical Professionals
page 379

Sources
page 383

PREFACE

It is odd the things one remembers.

Mother's hands were always delicate. Fine-boned and feminine, the fingernails free of polish. I cannot recall any adornment other than white-gold bands and the modest solitaire Dad bought with the first-prize money for his senior thesis.

My father's hands were long and strong, sinewy, the skin thicker and coarser than Mother's. As a child seated on his lap, with his arms wrapped around me, I would trace the dark hair along his wrists that disappeared under rolled-up shirtsleeves.

I grew accustomed to placing my hand in theirs in trust, or feeling their cool hands on my fevered brow.

Later I was touched with the sight of their hands entwined. How courtly it seemed when music would play, their eyes would meet, he'd reach out his hand, and they'd glide together into each other's arms.

Today when I think of those hands, they belong to thoughtful young adults wielding fountain pens and filling sheets of stationery. Seated at a desk in student quarters or a series of hospital wards, physicians in training Alice Baker of New Orleans and Joe Holoubek of Omaha opened their hearts and shared their passion for the healing profession. They wrote each other twice weekly as senior medical students and every day as interns.

In editing and researching their letters, I've had a rare privilege—getting to know my parents before they were parents, before they were even a couple. I like who they were as young people. I think we could have been friends.

Where once I was reluctant to read these letters, to intrude on their private moments, I now understand their immense social and historical value. My father and I started on this book together in the final months of his life. I offer it to the public in tribute to generations of high-minded health-care professionals and in testament to the truth of long-lasting love.

ALICE BAKER AND JOE HOLOUBEK met in 1937 during a summer fellowship program in pathology at Mayo Clinic. Only a few times would they meet again before marrying and starting their lives together in New Orleans.

Courting by letter launched a 65-year partnership—they were known affectionately as Dr. Alice and Dr. Joe—and helped shape groundbreaking careers. A graduate of Louisiana State University School of Medicine in New Orleans, Dr. Alice became one of the first women physicians to practice in northwest Louisiana, where they relocated after World War II. Dr. Joe, a University of Nebraska College of Medicine graduate and a consulting cardiologist, co-founded LSU School of Medicine in Shreveport.

The two became as widely known for their unbreakable bond as for their honors, achievements, and patient care. They worked together, worshipped together, raised four children, and never stopped dancing together—until silent strokes robbed her of short-term memory and frailty sapped the strength from his limbs.

This is the story of their courtship, drawn from a private collection of nearly 800 letters. It is a historical romance of considerable drama, reflecting the perils of medical training in the late 1930s and the social barriers challenging two-career marriages.

The letters, a treasure of primary source material, recreate the medical era before antibiotics, when tuberculosis ran rampant and health workers were at risk of serious infection. Overcrowding at New Orleans' Charity Hospital forced patients to share beds two or three at a time.

As interns, Dr. Alice, 23, and Dr. Joe, 22, set their sights on a return to Mayo Clinic, the medical mecca where they found each other and danced to the haunting "Harbor Lights." Grave illness and career setbacks shook their confidence, but they drew strength from the words of St. Paul: *Love endures . . . love never fails.* As the distant drumbeat of war grew closer, the two determined to face an uncertain future together, trusting in each other and the relationship they built letter by letter.

I am their youngest child, a former journalist and the editor of *Letters to Luke: From His Fellow Physician Joseph of Capernaum,* my father's last major accomplishment. The love and faith my parents shared inspired this gospel-based novel. Published in 2004, the award-winning work of fiction recounts in letters how a 1st century couple trained in the healing arts became friends and followers of Jesus.

At book signings, my father, then 88, charmed his audiences with the story of his courtship. They were delighted to learn the love letters still existed—boxes of yellowing envelopes preserved intact through several house moves and relocations. My father had recently organized them and had them bound—his letters to her and her letters to him—into eight volumes. My parents had begun rereading them and reliving their romance. They transported Mother, who could no longer keep the present within her grasp, to a time and place she remembered with joy.

The Courtship of Two Doctors began to take shape early in 2007, two years after Mother's death. It was then I suggested we have the letters transcribed, and we planned an abridged compilation of the collection. Sitting in his wheelchair before a desktop computer, my father wrote the first draft of a prologue. Set in Rochester, Minnesota, it would recount how they met.

For several months I probed his memory further and drew out more details. Where did you live that summer? How did you dress and what did you drive? What could you have said that so quickly piqued the interest of the girl from Louisiana? What did the two of you see or hear at Mayo Clinic that broadened your way of thinking and fueled your budding ambitions?

In answer to my questions, he unearthed a treasure I hadn't known existed: a five-year diary he kept during his medical training. It later proved invaluable in verifying facts and fleshing out the storyline of a summer seventy years past, allowing me access to private thoughts and feelings. I shall always cherish those journeys into my father's past, as he left us abruptly that year, at the age of 91, to rejoin his beloved Alice.

By that time, I was riveted by the historical content of the letters. I determined that, before tackling a condensed version, I would annotate all the transcribed letters and make them accessible to historians of health care and of academic medicine.

I traveled to Rochester, where the Mayo brothers' legacy of excellence continued to inspire young doctors, and to post-Katrina New Orleans, where the once grand and glorious Charity Hospital sat empty, silent, and shuttered. I also mined details from my father's other personal papers—memoirs and journal notations dating back to his childhood.

At St. Marys Hospital in Rochester, the delightful Sister Antoine Murphy R.N., then 93, shared still-vivid memories of late-1930s operating room and pathology lab procedures. In New Orleans, Russell C. Klein M.D., then associate dean for alumni affairs and development at LSU School of Medicine in New Orleans, generously offered material from his own book-in-progress, *A History of LSU School of Medicine New Orleans* (LSU Medical Alumni Association, 2010). I offer humble thanks to each of them; to Elsie Braswell, our painstaking and resourceful transcriptionist; and to my helpers in four states—librarians, historians, and archivists who helped supply missing first names and last names to the hundreds of people mentioned in the courtship letters. Their contributions enrich *The Holoubek-Baker Letters, 1937–1939: An Annotated Collection*, a two-volume compilation with 1,350 footnotes and twenty-four pages of research aids. Copies reside in medical and historical archives at LSU, the University of Nebraska, and Mayo Clinic.

Continuing my historical research, I explored the divergent philosophies of clinical training in 1930s Nebraska and Louisiana in the article "Courtship of Two Doctors: 1930s Letters Spotlight Nebraska Medical Training," *Nebraska History*, 92:2 (summer 2011). Medical students in Omaha started clinical service their sophomore year, learning how to take histories and make a physical diagnosis. As juniors, they took on hospital service. As seniors, they staffed outpatient clinics and made house calls throughout Omaha, shouldering an awesome amount of responsibility. In Louisiana, as at most U.S. medical schools, the two years of clinical training began junior year with outpatient clinic service. Seniors worked in hospital wards but had little autonomy.

Finally, I turned to the original book concept my father and I planned: a condensed version of the courtship correspondence. *The Courtship of Two Doctors* comprises excerpts from roughly 300 letters establishing the central storyline of classmates and pen pals whose fancy matures to love. My heartfelt thanks to Judy Pace Christie, novelist and former newspaper editor, who offered encouragement and constructive criticism on this project, much as she mentored me years ago in the newsroom of the Shreveport *Times*. And to my cousin Mary Baker Wood M.D., who provided invaluable research assistance, setting my wrongs aright on several technical aspects of medicine. For any remaining errors, I take full responsibility.

A note to historians: The letters were edited with a light hand, preserving the casual writing style and much of the archaic spelling and punctuation. I inserted first and last names where needed, corrected factual date errors, and made other changes for the sake of clarity, consistency, or readability. In editing the prologue, I relied on diary entries and fiction techniques to reconstruct events and conversations of seventy-five years ago.

A note to readers: The letters frequently crossed in the mail—that is, two or more arrived before an answer to the previous letter. No letters exist from Alice to Joe for eighteen days in January 1939. He was in Omaha's infectious diseases hospital, and letters he received were destroyed when he left, for fear of contamination. Lastly, I offer for your reference an outline of the medical training Alice and Joe received and an appendix with timeline and cast of characters—family, friends, and medical professionals.

May the story of Dr. Alice and Dr. Joe continue to inspire generations of young couples to cherish one another and build relationships based on mutual respect and high ideals.

May they rejoice in the journey of dreaming, living, and loving.

And may they forever be each other's safe havens and "Harbor Lights."

Martha Holoubek Fitzgerald
Shreveport, Louisiana
July 2012
www.marthafitzgerald.com

MEDICAL TRAINING

1937–1938, Senior year, medical school

Joe Holoubek
University of Nebraska College of Medicine, Omaha

Outcall (house call) duty all year
Additional appointment: Student physician,
    Nebraska Children's Home
Thesis due and completed on April 8 (wins first prize)
Dispensary services by semester:

FALL   Ophthalmology; obstetrics, gynecology, and newborn;
        allergy and tuberculosis

SPRING Urology; orthopedics; adult heart; dermatology and
        syphilology (treatment of syphilis); neurology; gastro-
        enterology; lab; ENT (ear, nose, and throat; also called
        oto-rhino-laryngology or ORL); pediatrics

M.D. awarded in June

Alice Baker
Louisiana State University School of Medicine,
    New Orleans

Ward work
Services by section:
    Internal medicine
    Obstetrics, gynecology, and newborn
    Pediatrics, tropical medicine, and neuro-psychiatry
    Surgery, urology, and orthopedics
Weekly medicine and surgery lectures, surgery diagnostic clinic
Clinical pathological conferences all year
B.M. awarded in June (M.D. awarded after internship)

1938–1939, general internships

Joe Holoubek
University Hospital, Omaha, 230 beds, 12 interns
(Training by rotating services rather than specialized or "straight service")

Services by month:
  July: Anesthetics
  August: Admitting room and NT (nose and throat)
  September: Obstetrics
  October: Gynecology
  November: Pediatrics and oral surgery
  December: Neurology, neurosurgery, psychiatry, and
      ophthalmology
  January: Orthopedics and urology (interrupted)
  February: Radiology and dermatology (delayed)
  March/April: Medicine
  May/June: Surgery

Alice Baker
Charity Hospital, New Orleans, 1,800 beds, 82 interns
(Last full year of operation; "new" Charity Hospital under construction)

Services by section:
  Tuberculosis, medicine, and dermatology
  Genito-urinary or G.U. (interrupted)
  Gynecology and obstetrics
  Surgery
  Ambulance duty (skipped)
  G.U. (resumed)

PROLOGUE

Rochester, Minnesota, 1937

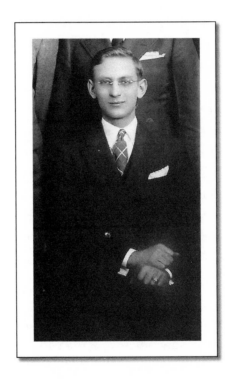

LOOKING BACK, I wasn't so favorably disposed toward Alice the day we met. When she first reported to MacCarty's lab, I turned to the other fellows in dismay. "There's a girl in the class!"

A hen medic.

Most every woman medical student I'd ever met sported short hair and slacks, as if she wanted to be one of the guys. Alice, it turned out, was different. She dressed neatly and handled herself like a lady. She had a soft Southern drawl. And she smiled a lot.

Now, five weeks later, our fellowship at Mayo Clinic is nearing its end, and so is our acquaintance. Alice will soon be but a pleasant memory of an exceptional summer. Just one of several girls whom I have met over the years, dated, and bid a quick farewell. Diversions, but little more.

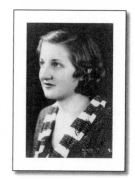

After all, we scarcely know one other. We've been out only four or five times—twice after staff meetings.

Still, she's a grand girl, this Alice Baker of New Orleans. What an accent!

And smart to boot.

Daughter of a doctor. A senior medical student, like me, a year away from a degree and internship. Only, Alice is being readied for big-city practice, while my training at the University of Nebraska aims to produce country doctors.

We are in Rochester as members of Dr. William Carpenter MacCarty's summer fellowship program in pathology. We attend lectures at his laboratory at St. Marys Hospital and observe firsthand his controversial method of specimen analysis.

"Uncle Mac," as we now call him, also philosophizes. "Progress is made by the minority," he says. "Be not afraid of criticism." He advises self-education and initiative. "Are we to be held back by the foolish traditions of the ancients?" Inspiring words—and good quotes for my growing collection.

Several of my friends in Omaha are pinned or engaged to girls back home, and my roommate got married four months ago. But I have no intention of settling down before I finish my internship. And maybe not even then. I'd like to see the world first. Perhaps I shall take postgraduate training in Austria, as did some of my professors—or in Czechoslovakia, my grandparents' homeland. I must admit, my ambitions have grown since I enrolled in medical school.

Besides, there is so much yet to learn—in the lecture halls at UN

College of Medicine, in the wards and clinics at University Hospital, on house calls across Omaha. This year I'll be busy running Nu Sigma Nu medical fraternity—the fellows just elected me president. I'll be student physician at an orphanage. And I still have a doctoral thesis to write. How grand that I may use the Mayo library while I'm here.

No, I did not come to Minnesota looking for romance.

Fascination. That's what this is. Fascination, nothing more.

"LECTURES USUALLY begin about the first of July," MacCarty wrote in his letter accepting me into the program, "but you may come as early as you like, to observe the routine surgical pathology." I arrived June 23.

Clarkson, my hometown in northeast Nebraska, is a day's drive from Rochester. I was accompanied by "A.C." Cimfel, junior medical student and my best friend since high school, who was headed on to Michigan for his own summer course.

A.C. and I are like brothers, especially since his parents died. His thick head of dark curls even reminds me of my mother's. I take after Father, with high cheekbones and blond hair that, to my dismay, is already thinning.

We checked in at the Kahler Hotel—three dollars a night, with a shared bath. The Kahler, which devotes two floors to surgical suites and hospital beds, connects to Mayo Clinic by means of tunnels. What a boon that must be during Minnesota winters.

That night in my diary, I jotted a quick note. *Ambition realized. I am in Rochester.*

Hard to believe, but I'd soon be rubbing elbows with students from Harvard, Dartmouth, and Tulane. I wondered if most of them would be doctors' sons, like many of the Nu Sigs.

My standing in Omaha had to have climbed a notch or two the day I won this fellowship.

In my mind, Mayo Clinic has no peer. It offers the best of care—everyone from the Midwest comes here when local doctors cannot help—and it places equal emphasis on research and training. "There are two objects of medical education," says Dr. Charlie Mayo, one of the founding brothers, "to heal the sick and to advance the science."

Most of what I know of Mayo's history I've learned since I arrived. This all started when Dr. Charlie, Dr. Will, and their father set up a group practice, one of the first of its kind. The three staffed Rochester's first hospital, St. Marys, which the Sisters of St. Francis opened in 1889. The brothers specialized in surgery. Their early adoption of antiseptic techniques cut down the risk of infection in patients, and word of the low patient death rate spread quickly. I learned that in 1905 they performed nearly four thousand operations.

Like their father, the younger Mayos traveled often and returned with new ideas about medicine. "The glory of medicine," Dr. Will once said, "is that it is constantly moving forward, that there is always more to learn."

The brothers invested their savings in a graduate education program in clinical medicine, associated with the University of Minnesota. They believed that excess earnings should return to the sick in the form of better-trained physicians—a noble thought—and placed physicians on salary. They created the Mayo Foundation for Medical Education and Research to run their clinic. It soon won national recognition, and Rochester swelled in size. *The Civic Weekly*, I see, reports a 1937 population of 23,000, with ten hospitals and sanitariums, four movie theaters, and forty-seven apartment houses.

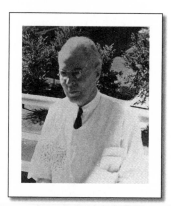

My first morning in town, A.C. and I walked to St. Marys Hospital, found MacCarty in the seven-story Surgical Pavilion, and introduced ourselves.

Dr. William Carpenter MacCarty at Mayo Clinic, 1937

MacCarty showed us his laboratory, the operating room suites, and the surgical amphitheater, which can seat 200 observers. Before A.C. left to catch his train, he and I watched one operation from the gallery. The rest of the hospital I explored on my own. Enlarged half a dozen times, St. Marys is a rambling facility with 600 patient beds.

I discovered a large chapel with vaulted ceiling, marble floors, and corridors wide enough for people in wheelchairs and hospital carts. A golden light bathed the aisles. I sat in the quiet for some time, enjoying the same sense of a higher being that I feel in the cathedral in Omaha.

Finally, I returned downtown and sought out Mayo's library. It's on the 12th floor of the 1928 Plummer Building, a soaring structure of limestone and brick that commands downtown Rochester. Floodlit at night, the Plummer's bell tower casts an inviting beam deep into the darkness over southeastern Minnesota.

In the library's reading room, marble arches drew my glance upward to the oak ceiling. It's embellished with gilt and green paint. Inscribed on beams 17 feet above are the names of dozens of physicians and scientists. Lavoisier. Osler. Lister. Curie. Pasteur. . . .

I looked around and took a deep breath, committing to memory the handsome room, the reverent hush, and the tantalizing smell of leather-bound books promising untold riches of knowledge. Here, I knew, was where I would spend most of my evenings.

I introduced myself to the librarian on duty and was elated to hear the research materials were at my disposal. Now I could write a good senior thesis. The subject is climate—that is, the effect of the climate on health. It's a topic of great interest to my dean, Dr. C.M. W. Poynter, who also chairs the anatomy department. He helped Nebraska's College of Medicine consolidate from two campuses to one—in Omaha—in 1913.

How well I remember my first day of medical school. Dean Poynter greeted the freshman class with an edict. "Gentlemen, as of this day you are members of a distinguished profession. I expect never to see you out of proper dress—a suit and tie." And so it has been for three years.

I found a room with the Keily family on 1st Street SW, between the hospital and the clinic. The household includes three girls of high school age. They remind me of the boarders my mother takes in back home—farm girls who arrive every Sunday afternoon and go home after school on Fridays.

As the other summer fellows turned up in Rochester, I acted as welcoming committee. I greeted them in MacCarty's lab and showed them around the hospital. That is, until Alice appeared, and then Mary Giffin, a pre-med student at Smith College whose father was Mayo chief of staff.

So women claimed two of the spots in the summer fellowship program.

I let them find their own way around.

Later, after my first evening with Alice, I would regret my rudeness.

On Wednesday nights, we were privileged to attend staff meetings. The papers presented were published and widely disseminated in the medical world as *Proceedings of the Staff Meetings of the Mayo Clinic.*

One week into our course, I took a seat in Plummer Hall and prepared to take detailed notes. Until that day I had exchanged few words with the girl student from Louisiana. But that was about to change.

The meeting started promptly at 8:15 p.m. as the summer sun, pouring in through the bank of leaded-glass windows, lost its grip on the day. I admired the grand setting—an oak-paneled assembly area that claimed two upper floors of the Plummer Building. Equipped with stereopticons, motion-picture equipment, and theater-style seating, Plummer Hall accommodates an audience of 250. It was full that night. The special guest, hearing reports on gastric carcinoma and low-potassium diets, was the First Lady herself, Eleanor Roosevelt.

Only thirty minutes into the presentation, however, I began to wilt under my suit coat. July nights could be sweltering, even in Minnesota. A drying wind from the south had chased away June's rain, delivering several days of high-mercury temperatures that hung on past nightfall. I needed some air.

I slipped out with the first members of the audience, as the meeting drew to a close, and entered the first bronze-fitted elevator. Moments later Mrs. Roosevelt, trailed by assistants, swept out of the hall into the lobby. As she moved toward the bank of elevators, the throng of physicians, professors, researchers, and students parted to make way. "Hold the door for the First Lady!"

I stepped back and hunched my shoulders, aiming to separate the starched shirt from the small of my back. The elevator cage soon filled, with a second woman stepping in at the last moment. Mrs. Roosevelt's diamond rings flashed in the artificial light, but it wasn't the First Lady who held my attention. It was the other woman— Alice Baker.

A thought occurred to me between floors. *If I ask out a girl from the South, won't the Nu Sigs be impressed!*

Moments later, the elevator door opened. Mrs. Roosevelt's entourage strode out through the first-floor lobby and down a short flight of stairs to the street. I caught up with Alice, matching my longer stride to her purposeful steps.

"Hot night, isn't it, Alice?" I didn't wait for her answer. "Would you like to take a drive to cool off? I'll introduce you to Nellie."

Alice gave me a sidelong glance, slowing her pace. "Who's Nellie?" She paused outside the towering bronze entry doors, letting others rush past us. I worried a moment that she'd turn me down, then saw her eyes blink and the flicker of a smile cross her brow. "Sure, Joe. I was just going to walk the couple of blocks home, but thank you."

I guided Alice across the street and stopped before a 1934 Model A sedan.

"This is Nellie."

She laughed.

"It's my father's car. Mine's back in Nebraska getting an overhaul. It's a 1928 Studebaker Commander. I call her Nancy."

Alice grinned, as if she enjoyed the wit. She stepped to Nellie's side and let me open the door for her. In the glow of the streetlamp, I took notice of her fair skin and wavy brown hair. Her blue eyes held my green ones for just a moment longer than necessary.

I shed my jacket and laid it on the rear seat. Popping open Nellie's vent windows to catch the breeze, I drove Alice through town. We stopped at a drive-in, sipped 5-cent Coca-Colas, and talked about MacCarty and our course of study.

From the first day, MacCarty challenged the teachings of our medical schools regarding the diagnosis of cancer. The standard method of specimen analysis, using frozen tissue, was not effective, he taught, in spotting early-stage cancer.

As the day's round of surgeries began in the ten operating rooms, surgeons would place specimens of gastric ulcers on a plate and send them to MacCarty to analyze for malignancies. They then awaited his pathology report before deciding how much of a patient's stomach to remove.

In fewer than five minutes, while we watched, MacCarty would cut sections of tissue, stain them, place the slides under his double-vision microscope—a binocular, it's called—analyze them, and send his report down the hall.

Sometimes he would meet with the family of the patient to discuss the probable prognosis.

Then he would invite us to look through the binocular ourselves and see how tissues looked during an actual operation, before they were changed through a fixation process. The nucleolus within the nucleus, he showed us, is larger in a cancerous cell than in a healthy cell.

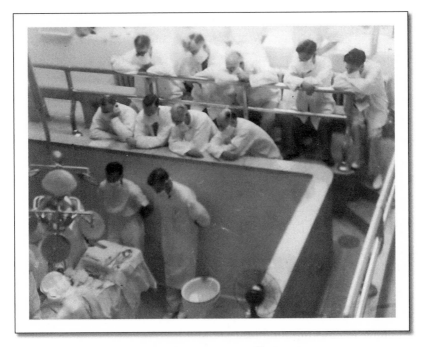

Observing surgery, Mayo Clinic, 1937

For the rest of the day, we were free to observe operations, attend clinics, and join hospital rounds. It was a chance to observe some of the best physicians in the country at work—among them, Dr. Russell Wilder in endocrinology, Dr. Philip S. Hench in rheumatology, and Dr. J. Arnold Bargen in gastro-enterology. Dr. Wilder had conducted one of the first clinical trials of insulin.

MacCarty would encourage us to see as much as we could. "Go!" he said. "This is why you are here! See something you would not see at school."

And wherever I went—clinics at Curie Hospital, surgeries and ward rounds at St. Marys—I would encounter Alice.

One day, Dr. Hench described the analgesic effect of jaundice and hepatitis on rheumatoid arthritis—that is, patients experienced a lessening of their chronic pain. He and his assistants had devised an experimental treatment to transfuse jaundiced blood into an arthritic, trying it first on rabbits. Another day, we watched the chief neurosurgeon, Dr. Alfred W. Adson, operate.

Alice and I laughed, recalling the scene. All we could see from the gallery was the back of his head, but we could hear well. Dr. Adson grew agitated and bawled out everyone in the operating room, even the Sisters of St. Francis who were assisting.

"I would not want to cross Dr. Adson," Alice remarked.

"Nor would I!"

Then there was the day we met Dr. Will and Dr. Charlie Mayo. Still active as surgical consultants, they dropped by MacCarty's pathology lab. They seemed to be just regular fellows, Alice said, and I agreed. They did not put on airs.

By the time I drove Alice home and walked her to the door—she was staying with Mary Lomasney, a social worker whose family once lived in Louisiana—I was intrigued.

"So, Alice," I asked abruptly, "may I take you to the Giffins' lawn party next Wednesday?"

"Oh!" Alice caught her breath. There it was again—something in her eyes. A hesitancy. A bit of shyness perhaps. Then her face seemed to light up from within. "Thank you, Joe. I'd like that!"

As I turned back toward Nellie, I couldn't help smiling.

THE DAY ARRIVED for the lawn party. Nellie was washed and shined and ready for the evening. I put on my white linen suit, white shoes, and black tie. When Alice opened her door, she was wearing a simply cut dress. I liked the way it swirled around her legs.

We drove to the Giffin home on Eighth Avenue SW and joined the other summer fellows chatting with our professors, local physicians, and several post-graduate fellows. I looked for my friend Ivan Rutledge, a recent Nebraska graduate and fellow Nu Sig.

Dinner was laid out on long, cloth-covered tables on the Giffin lawn. There was lively debate over the merits of sulfanilamide—trade names prontylin and prontosil—the new wonder drug for infections of all kinds. And dismay at the prospect of federalized health care. The issue had dominated discussion at June's American Medical Association meeting in Atlantic City.

Alice and Mary, I noticed, drew a good bit of attention as the only girls in our group. They both handled themselves well, even taking unpopular stands for the sake of argument.

"Perhaps if the government controlled medical care," Alice said, "poor people could afford better treatment. And doctors would get their bills paid on time."

"Good points," I countered, "but I'm still against it. We don't need pencil pushers getting in the way when we talk to our patients." And so it went, pro and con, with the girls holding their own in every conversation.

Finally, Alice and I took our leave. I drove her to Silver Lake, a new park that opened earlier in the summer. I had been swimming there, and I enjoyed the view of the city from the north shore. As dusk fell, the Plummer Building's bell tower began to glow like the first star of the night.

We sat in the car listening to big band music on the radio. To my surprise, Alice seemed as interested in my family history as I was in hers.

For Alice, I learned, medicine was a high calling and a family tradition. Her father, an Indiana native who trained in Louisville, Kentucky, is now a chest specialist at a veterans hospital in Pineville, Louisiana, outside Alexandria. Her brother in New York is a doctor and her sister in Virginia a nurse. There have been doctors in the Baker family since the War of 1812.

Alice attends LSU School of Medicine in New Orleans, now in its sixth year.

I soon realized how little I knew about Louisiana. Everyone back home assumed Southerners were slow and somewhat ignorant. Then there was Louisiana's shady governor, Huey Long, the populist who wanted to be president. "Say, wasn't he elected to the Senate and then assassinated in his own state capitol?"

"Yes, Joe. It was horrible." Alice stared straight ahead into the gathering darkness. "It was two years ago last September, and they said it was a doctor who killed him. Our dean tried to save his life." Alice's chin rose and she turned her head, pulling my glance to hers.

"But Joe, it was Huey Long who started LSU's medical school. He knew Louisiana needed doctors to treat all the poor people, and not everyone could afford to go to Tulane. He insisted we get some of the best professors in the country. Within two years, LSU was rated a Class A medical school."

And now, Alice told me, the state is building a splendid new public hospital in New Orleans on the site of the old one. The new Charity will be the second largest hospital in the country with 2,680 beds. "They say it will have 50 operating rooms and need more than 150 residents, from LSU, Tulane, and elsewhere. Already we call it Charity the Beautiful."

Alice sighed. "I hope it opens soon. Conditions are horribly over-crowded now. They're tearing down some of the 100-year-old build-ings to make room for the new one, and patients in many wards have to share a bed. Most of the Negro wards have been moved down the street to the old Pythian Temple."

I retrieved a pack of Old Golds from my coat pocket, tapped out two cigarettes, and offered Alice a smoke. She accepted. Her hands, I noticed, were delicate and free of jewelry. There were no nicotine stains on her fingers.

"So, Alice," I asked, "when did you decide to become a doctor?"

"At LSU in Baton Rouge." She leaned forward as I lit her cigarette. "My parents did not want me to study medicine. 'It's a hard life for a woman,' they said."

But she persisted, inspired in part by her father. Dr. E.S. Baker started out as a country doctor. Mother Baker taught music and assisted in his horse-and-buggy practice. In 1910 they moved from Indiana to Arkansas, and in 1917, at age 47, he joined the U.S. Army Medical Corps. Discharged after Armistice with a weak heart, he left private practice and turned to government service. He took graduate training in lung diseases at Tulane University School of Medicine in New Orleans before accepting the first of a series of assignments to veterans hospitals.

Alice's father and mother made themselves at home wherever they were posted, joining the Methodist church, the Masonic lodge, and the Order of the Eastern Star. For the past nine years, they'd lived in a house on the hospital grounds in Pineville, along with ailing Aunt Mary Baker, formerly a head nurse.

Dr. Baker—now a ward surgeon nearing retirement—treated patients with tuberculosis.

"TB is taking a terrible toll on veterans," Alice said. "It's a slow way to die." She looked at the half-smoked Old Gold in her hand, shook her head, and crushed it out in Nellie's ashtray. "We see a lot of it in New Orleans. There must be a thousand more patients who need treatment than our hospitals can handle."

Her eyes grow clouded. "My brother's wife has tuberculosis. Marie is in and out of sanitariums, and Ray has to raise their two children. I wish I could do more to help."

"So, Joe," she said, smoothing the dress on her lap and changing the subject, "have you decided where you want to intern?"

"No, not yet," I replied, stubbing out my own cigarette. "I started medical school intending to be a small-town doctor, but now I'm not so sure. You're making Charity Hospital sound very appealing."

Alice settled back to hear the rest of my story.

I was born on a farm near Clarkson, a town of about 800 in the hills of eastern Nebraska.

My father used a horse and single plow to break the ground each year for spring planting. When I was too young to be of much help, I enjoyed walking behind him, barefoot in the freshly plowed earth.

Both my parents were first-generation Americans raised in sod houses—prairie homes built of the soil their fathers tilled as homesteaders. And until I started school, I spoke only Czech, the language of my Bohemia-born grandparents.

My father left farming when his lungs were weakened by influenza. Now he runs the Clarkson oil station. He's one of only two Catholic business owners in town. "I have worked with him every summer since I was twelve," I said.

"Money is tight these days, but the filling station is holding its own. People still have to drive. When they cannot pay for their gasoline, he puts it on the books. Dad works late into the night and on weekends—but he loves to laugh, play cards, and pull pranks on people.

"I have one sister. She taught school before marrying a farmer. Louis is a fine fellow. Gosh, their baby is due soon—Sept. 1—and we are all a bit concerned. Adela's first child, a little girl, was stillborn."

"Oh, Joe, how sad."

"Well, everything seems to be OK this time. But if Adela needs it, we will bring her to Omaha for a specialist's care.

"You know," I said, leaning forward, "my father was disappointed when I decided to study medicine. He hoped that I would take over his business. But Mother was pleased. She had dreamed of being a nurse, but had to leave school to keep house for a bachelor brother."

I fell silent for a moment, watching the light at the Clinic blink across the water and remembering my first days away from home. I started college in Lincoln at age 16. A.C. and I shared a room at a boarding house a block from campus. Tuition was $30 a semester. I mailed shirts home every week in a metal box with black straps. Mother returned them in the next post, cleaned, starched, and pressed.

"The wife of the Clarkson doctor told my mother that I would never make it through medical school—I was just an oilman's son. That hurt," I said, avoiding Alice's gaze.

"I resolved to work harder and make better grades than my schoolmates, and got accepted to the College of Medicine after two years of study. I waited tables at the NΣN house my sophomore year, for spending money. Tuition is $250 a semester. I hate to think how hard my dad has to work to keep me in school," I said, shifting in my seat to look Alice in the eye. "And now Mother worries I will not find a good place to practice. Country doctors are having a hard time making ends meet."

I sat back again and sighed. "I'm being trained for general practice, but I now know that will not satisfy me. I hope to master at least one field of medicine. Maybe I shall be a researcher and educator, like Uncle Mac."

Alice smiled. "You'd be a good teacher, Joe." She leaned toward me and placed her hand on my arm. "You could do whatever you set your mind to."

I paused for a moment, enjoying her closeness. "I do hope you're right. I have learned to make the acquaintance of anyone who can help me achieve my goals. That is one reason I joined the fraternity."

I smiled. "You know, they are a grand bunch of fellows. It was a Nu Sig who told me about MacCarty's fellowship program. The father of another helped me apply. Now, as the new chapter president, I may be able to help others get ahead.

"But I must focus on my speaking skills. They're lousy. Whenever I have to lead a meeting or address a gathering, I write out my remarks ahead of time and memorize them. I stammer," I confessed to Alice, somewhat to my surprise.

"Joe, I never noticed that. . . . And I so much admire you for being president. Gee, based on what I've seen with my sorority, that must be a lot of hard work."

Alice was helping organize a New Orleans chapter of a medical sorority. "We'll be so excited when Alpha Epsilon Iota accepts us."

In every other campus group, Alice said, she and her friends were among the minority. Since the day they'd enrolled at the medical school, the girls had endured a lot of razzing. But it was mostly in good fun, she said. "We get along pretty well with the boys."

These days, her parents are among her biggest supporters, and several of her father's Veterans Hospital colleagues had rallied behind her.

"It was Dr. Will O'Daniel Jones, the surgical chief, who encouraged me to apply here at Mayo," Alice said. "He's also let me scrub in for surgery.

"Dr. Jones thinks I should apply for a graduate fellowship here once I finish in New Orleans. It would mean one year each of hospital, laboratory, and clinical experience. Oh, Joe, wouldn't that be grand?"

I had to admire the grit behind her smile. It was easily as strong as my own resolve. Alice, only two semesters from a medical degree, didn't intend to let anyone hold her back just because she was a woman.

THE NEXT FEW DAYS, I found several occasions to sit beside Alice—in the lecture hall, at the binocular in the laboratory, in the operating room galleries. She asked difficult questions, and I could tell our classmates were developing respect for her mind.

I had been spending time with several of the other fellows, double-dating to picnics and picture shows, or just going out for a beer, but I began to find their company less satisfying.

I have never enjoyed rowdy parties. If someone tries to force me to do something against my will, I am more determined not to do it. I want to be able, as the days go by, to look myself straight in the eyes.

And I tend to grow silent in large groups. Fifteen years after learning English, I still fret over my grammar, and the proper words often elude me.

With Alice, however, I conversed as easily as with the girls back home. And we laughed often.

I told her there's a woman doctor in Nebraska I know and admire—Dr. Olga Stastny, also of Czech descent. She's from a small town near Clarkson and finished medical school in 1912. Trained as a surgeon, she did relief work after the war in Czechoslovakia, Greece, and Turkey. Now she lives and works in Omaha, practicing obstetrics and gynecology.

"I should like to meet her one day," Alice said. She and her roommate Dorothy Mattingly, the sister of a physician, enjoy meeting the women doctors in New Orleans.

"Say, what did you think of Uncle Mac's statement this morning?" I asked. "He claimed he had no love for money. He's either a true scientist or a big windbag."

Alice laughed softly. "He does have a big ego. But he certainly could be making more money if he were somewhere else, in private practice. I admire him for that."

"Do you remember," I asked, "when he described the different stages of life? He dubbed the years between 45 and 55 the Age of Wisdom...."

"And he can't be much more than 55 himself," Alice said, finishing my thought. "No doubt he changes that age bracket as he himself grows older!"

"No doubt, indeed," I said with a smile. "But Uncle Mac has a point. At this stage in our lives, we must pick out the characteristics of those whom we admire and make them our own."

"How true. But Joe, we'll have to refrain from quoting him so much once we return to school! Most professors don't like to be challenged."

And with that thought, Alice and I arranged to meet at the next staff meeting. The program would include a cardiac clinic—how to manage and treat coronary thrombosis. But I had a longer evening in mind.

"Would you like to go dancing afterward?" I asked. "The Valencia Ballroom has an orchestra." I was fairly confident on the ballroom floor, having danced the polka since I was a boy. There are dances every Sunday night in Clarkson, and a ballroom in nearby Howells brings in orchestras.

"I'd love to," Alice said, her cheeks coloring slightly.

How sweet she looks when she blushes, I thought.

The next Wednesday, once the staff meeting ended, I drove Alice to the Valencia, on the west side of town. The ballroom, lined with tables and booths, had a mirrored chandelier that revolved.

I paid a dollar for two tickets and took Alice to the dance floor for the first time. The tune was "Josephine." She easily responded to my lead. And she fit nicely in my arms, just about five inches shorter than my six feet.

The next week, I took Alice to the Pla-Mor dance hall on the south side of town. We favored waltzes and fox trots. On Friday evening, we attended another lawn party, this time at the home of Dr. MacCarty. His son Collin was a summer fellow. And on Sunday we went for a drive in the country.

Alice admired my 35 mm camera—she had a Brownie at home— but ducked my efforts to snap her picture. "You'll break your camera!"

"Argus can take it," I said, using another pet name. "I paid $4.25 for this beauty last year—I have a friend who bought it for me wholesale. And I'm learning how to develop the film myself."

By the day the summer fellows' class picture was taken, on the lawn outside St. Mary's Hospital, it only seemed natural that I take my place beside Alice.

I'm the one dressed in white.

So HERE WE ARE, in the first week of August. Only one week of lectures remains. Alice will leave for home immediately—it's a two-day bus ride to "Alex," as she calls it—but I plan to stay several more days.

Tonight may be our last dance date, so I've brought Alice back to the Valencia.

On the ballroom floor, I put aside all thoughts of the future. Only the present matters.

And Alice feels so good in my arms.

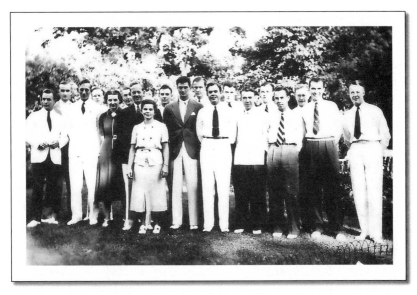

Members of summer fellowship program in pathology, Mayo Clinic, 1937. Joe Holoubek is third from left and Alice Baker is standing beside him.

She seems to sense my moves before I make them. I sweep her in ever-more confident circles across the floor, surrendering to the music and the mood and the moment.

We dance until the music trails off. Alice laughs and rubs the side of her face as I lead her off the floor. "My cheeks hurt from smiling!"

Unwilling to call it a night, we drive to Silver Lake and sit in the car at the overlook. More big band sounds pour from the radio, which picks up stations from across the Midwest.

Then "Harbor Lights" plays—the British hit has become one of our favorite songs—and I grow pensive.

> *I saw the harbor lights*
> *They only told me we were parting*
> *The same old harbor lights that once brought you to me. . . .*

With Alice's hand in mine, I imagine the city lights across the lake are the harbor lights of New Orleans, and we are together on the banks of the Mississippi, enjoying a soft breeze off the water.

But no, I tell myself. *No, this is not to be.*

This romance could never last.

Omaha and New Orleans are 1,100 miles apart.

Our cultures are different. Our families are different. Our religions are different.

Surely, I tell myself, *Alice has finer suitors in New Orleans. Doctors' sons, not farm boys.*

The mood broken, I start the car, drive Alice home, and steel myself to say a casual goodnight. I don't call for her on Sunday, spending most of the day working on my thesis.

The last few days of the fellowship pass quickly. On Thursday night, I walk over to Alice's apartment to say goodbye, but spend as much time talking with Mary as with Alice.

I ask for Alice's mailing address in Louisiana, but make no promises I cannot keep.

I do not offer to drive her to the bus station on Friday.

The romance, such as it was, has ended. It was fascination, nothing more.

ONE

SENIOR YEAR
Nebraska & Louisiana

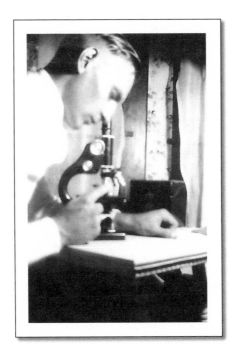

'I have never met a girl like you'

August–September 1937

⟨⟩

Dear Alice:

I hope that you forgive me for this tardy letter, but I have been very busy since I came home last Monday. Incidentally, I became an uncle Thursday and everything was normal this time—quite a relief.

I was rather surprised to come to Nebraska and find the corn fields dry. Quite a contrast to Minnesota.

Did you have a nice trip back? And how is Mary enjoying her trip to Mexico? I'll send her the kolache recipe when she gets back to Rochester.

Incidentally, Dr. MacCarty and Dr. Wilder got into quite a dispute about Pernicious Anemia, etc., last week and can they get mad. It was fun to have a ringside seat.

Knute Foster said that he sent you pictures. I hope that you received them by now. I printed a roll of mine, so I am enclosing a few. Will send more later.

Thanks for the folder of Louisiana. I think my next trip (internship) should be to the South.

Sincerely,

Joe

Alexandria
U.S. Veterans Hospital
Friday, Sept. 3

Dear "Uncle Joe"—

And how is the new niece/nephew or both? A remarkable child, I know, especially if he lives up to his uncle. I suppose I too should begin with an apology for my lateness in answering, but my days have been rather full. My sister and 3½ year old niece kept me occupied until I took them to New Orleans and put them on the train—and on the way back I convinced my roommate, Dot, to come home with me. She just left.

I did appreciate your letter and the picture so much—and just when did you snap that one of me? Don't you know the life of a candid camera man is full of danger? And—pretty please—I'd like so much a better picture of you. The one I got from Foster didn't half do you justice.

Isn't it inconsiderate of the "authorities" to open school so early? I haven't had enough time at home to be anxious for it to start yet. Ours starts the 13th, after which time my address will be 116 So. Johnson St., New Orleans. And all letters will be truly welcome as I'm trying "living alone and liking it" for the first time.

I haven't heard from Mary since her arrival, so I suppose she's OK. And aren't you going to let me in on those recipes?

Just
Alice

CLARKSON

Tuesday, Sept. 7

Dearest Alice:

I was very pleased to receive your letter and I must answer it before I leave for school. Incidentally, my fraternity has acquired a new house this year, so we have to be in Omaha Sept. 10th to prepare for fall rush week.

You mention a photograph of myself. I am not in the habit of posing for portraits, and the results are poor. However, I will send you one that my mother and I made last week. It is the best that I have. As you see, I cannot get my own camera to lie about my features and make me presentable.

Yes, life is never safe for a candid camera man—but, gee, isn't it fun to be in danger most of the time? And yes, I felt that way B.M. (before MacCarty), so my summer did not influence that idea any.

Incidentally, have you realized how much trouble some of Dr. MacCarty's ideas may bring to us in examinations? Nevertheless, I still believe some of them and will argue with anyone.

I will send some of the recipes. I found an old Bohemian cookbook, and with the help of my mother, I will try to translate them.

My nephew Dennis is certainly imitating me now—always crying and howling like I did. My address will be 4102 Farnam St., Omaha, and I do enjoy your letters.

And may I have a portrait of you, too.

As ever,

Joe

NEW ORLEANS
116 So. Johnson
Saturday, Sept. 18

My dear Joe—

You just can't imagine how very much good your letter did me. It seems that about everything bad which could possibly happen did happen, and all within the last two weeks. First we got a wire from my brother that his wife was critically ill and not expected to live, so Mother went at once to New York to be with them— and their 2 children.

At the same time, Dot scared us to death by having "almost" a heart attack. And in the midst of my packing for school, an aunt, two uncles and a niece popped in unexpectedly. We had a grand visit, but I'm still discovering things I forgot to pack.

I had just come back from registering in N.O. so I could spend all the time I could at home with Dad and Aunt Mary when I got your letter—and recipes—and, best of all, your picture. Now that I've told my sob story and been sympathized with, I'm sure (just like the baby of a family I can hear you say), let me thank you for them. Your mother must be an excellent photographer as well as cook. No, it doesn't flatter you at all, but I find myself wanting to talk to and get better acquainted with that nice looking boy of whose picture I'm the proud possessor.

Do you mind if I rave a bit if I promise I mean every word of it? You see, I'd never met anyone who had such truly fine and clean ideas and thoughts and ambitions before, and what's more, I know you are going to live up to them. Of course, my dad was in that niche, but I'm so glad to know a younger man who has all that now to help him mold his life as he meets it.

Oh dear, I'm so afraid that sounds utterly sickening and silly, but I'm not used to putting things like that which I feel into words. I suppose what I'm really trying to say is that I'm glad I got to meet you in Rochester and I'm proud of the picture.

Now, forgive me that and let me tell you about school. We have a new dean, Dr. J.R. D'Aunoy, and we're all pretty petrified of him. Already, our class has had a blow. Three boys conditioned surgery and had to take a make-up exam this week. Only one boy passed it. We suppose that means they'll have to repeat it and thus lose a year.

I suppose I'd better warn you that all I think about—and, it seems, all I write about after the middle of September—is school, school, school. So if you have enough of that already, don't mind hushing me up in the early stages. By the way, Ellanor Lockhart, one of the girl interns, is now in the hospital with TB. Terrible, isn't it?

I'm anxious to try those recipes, but maybe it's best I didn't get a chance to with Mother gone. I might have had a lot of explaining to do—Ha. I only have, now, a photograph taken two years ago, and I may have changed since then. What do you think?

I'm hoping to hear from you, if this hasn't been too much.

Alice

Omaha
4102 Farnam
Sunday, Sept. 26

Dearest Alice:

The past two weeks have been the busiest that I have ever spent in Omaha. My fraternity moved to a different house, which necessitated much extra work. After that we discarded our roles as painters, carpenters, and furniture movers and did some very active rushing, with the results of a fine pledge class. Now we are starting to school for a vacation—at least, it seems like a rest after our previous hard work.

My senior work is very interesting—have most of my time taken up with dispensaries. I happen to be student physician at the Nebraska Children's Home, so that places me on outcall duty all year. I will start on Obstetrics outcall next week.

We had quite a surprise last Friday when the instructor in Metabolism announced an examination on history of Metabolism. Now I wish that I had listened more closely during his lectures.

Fortunately, we have not lost anyone from our class yet. About 4 sophs and 4 freshmen have to repeat the year.

You mention your troubles. I am glad that you did. Your letter came at a time when I thought that I had some, but they were nothing compared to yours. However, we are all fortunate compared to my roommate, who received the news that his father died this forenoon. We hope from the bottom of our hearts that he will be able to return to school this year. Which proves that we never know what the future holds in store for us.

Two extremes—Lavoisier says "Life is a chemical function" while others say "Life is a series of hard knocks and disappointments." However, we must remember Longfellow's words, "Behind the clouds, the sun is still shining." Let us try to practice this even though it is unusually difficult sometimes.

Considering the future—well-made plans often are destroyed by unforeseen incidents, but I will still continue to do what I think best.

And now, the past, particularly this summer. We all made a multitude of new friendships and acquaintances and were impressed by numerous individuals. As time passes on, however, only a few of these friendships persist and the others remain as only memories. Allow me to say that I treasure my friendship with you above any others that I made this summer. It is extremely rare that anyone gets to meet a girl like you, with such pleasing manners, a wonderful personality, high morals, high intellectual training, and above all a good cook. The medical profession is fortunate to have you as one of its members. The treasured moments that we spent together have now passed into eternity, but the memories return to me daily. Frankly, I have never met a girl like you and I do hope that we can meet again sometime. Until then, we must content ourselves by exchanging our ideas and thoughts by letter.

I hope that your sister-in-law is better now and your father is well.

Duty calls now—a rushee is coming up and I must work for Nu Sigma Nu.

Write soon please.

> Love,
> Joe

'I had better quit philosophizing'

October–December 1937

My dearest Joe—

I am so glad that my newest patient presented a fairly typical picture so I could finish with her care early and have time to write to you tonight. This is the reward I bribed myself with to make me finish my work first! Your letter, which was so understanding, brought me good luck, for my sister-in-law is so much better and Mother will be in N. Orleans on her way home tomorrow. May I add my sincere wishes that your roommate may continue his school year.

Long live Nu Sigma Nu! I'm sure it will, as long as its members—and Presidents—are as active as those of your chapter. Now I'll have to brag a bit. Alpha Epsilon Iota has initiated a very active member of the surgery faculty, and she's hoping to get national recognition. Is your favorite doctor of the "weaker" sex the member of a national sorority?

Every once in a while I find myself starting to disagree with some professor, basing my argument on one of Dr. MacCarty's theories. Luckily, I've caught myself in time. I'd love to see the expression on our Clinical Path professor's face if I told him what Dr. Mac said about the way we study blood. However, I don't want to see it badly enough to risk his ire—and the grade he might give me. Oh, the injustices of the present educational system!

One of the boys in my class spent the summer in Greenville, Miss., at the Gamble Clinic. Do you remember Lyne Gamble from the summer group? His uncle and father, I believe, really have a wonderful clinic. It must be nice to have such a future prepared for you.

You really must be busy working now. Is your work at the Children's Home an extra job, or a part of your school work? I haven't been called on a home OB case as yet but am expecting a call at anytime, as I am second on the list. I gave my first anesthetic Thurs. p.m. and was so scared that I think my state of shock was worse than the patient's. However, we both survived and are getting along nicely.

I suppose that if I want to believe all those nice things you said about me I'd better learn to be a good cook—because that discrepancy is so great it will have to be overcome. Of course, there is a discrepancy about the others too, but I'd like to believe you meant part of what you wrote, at least. So just come see us soon and I promise you kolaches and coffee. Notice I don't say how good they'll taste though.

Oh, there seem to be so many experiences I'd like to share with you! For instance, the moment when I found out that the juice of six lemons a day will positively cure a case of pellagra. It honestly gave me a funny thrilling feeling, for I have a patient now, 17 years old, an LSU student, with an early case and over whose prospects I had been lamenting. We've been seeing so many autopsies on incurable or wrongly diagnosed cases that to know you can give true relief and cure by your own knowledge and power makes you know you have chosen the right profession.

Yes, the silver lining has shown through for me. I hope it is shiny and bright for you and remains so. How about polishing the lining to my cloud with another letter soon?

Love,
Alice

OMAHA

Tuesday, Oct. 5

Dearest Alice:

We just had a midnight lunch of kolaches that I brought from home Sunday. They were a little dry but still very tasty.

My roommates are having a grand time discussing the instructors—I bet that a few ears are ringing now. However, a few of the professors might profit by hearing of their faults. In fact, we all would and I like people who tell me mine rather than talk behind my back.

I am listening to "Harbor Lights," my favorite number. Could we dance it together at the Valencia again? Or perhaps somewhere else.

This past weekend has been hilarious in Omaha and Lincoln due to the fact that Neb. beat Minn. for the first time in over twenty years.

However, I spent a rather quiet weekend due to the death of my uncle from pulmonary embolism. Medical science has advanced with such great studies, but still there are some conditions over which we have no control. In other words, there is still so much for us to do in the future, and I hope that someone develops a successful treatment for this. Why not one of us? Are you interested?

You mention OB home delivery. I have had two already. What a thrill to bring a new life into this world. That is what makes medicine so fascinating for me—a new experience and thrill with every patient.

Internships and thesis are my great concerns now. Charity in New Orleans is practically closed to outsiders. Peter Bent Brigham Hospital in Boston is a straight service, and so are most of the other Eastern hospitals. Where do you plan to go? I am planning a fellowship at Mayo's eventually. Are you going there?

My friend Dr. Rutledge from the Clinic is visiting here now, so that brings me a little nearer to my summer memories.

You may wonder why this is such a long letter, but I have so much to say. And I do like to hear all about you and your work.

I must close and get some needed sleep, but I would rather write to you.

I plan to write to Dr. MacCarty tomorrow and praise his course again. Will that help his ego?

Love,
Joe

NEW ORLEANS
Sunday, Oct. 10

Dear Joe—

Again I'm bribing myself. There's only one thing I'd rather do than write to you, it seems, and that is to get a letter from you. And as far as your faults go, the only ones I can think of are that you live too far away and you've given me a "yardstick" to measure people by that no one else I've met seems to measure up to. You take your sorrows and turn them into inspirations and ambitions. May you continue to make all of these develop into realizations.

And you've also beat me at the stork game. I've only delivered one baby, but such a cute one that I like to make my postpartal calls so I can play with her. She's halfway a namesake of mine, too, even though her mother did think I looked rather young to be helping her baby into the world. The actual delivery turns out to be quite different from "book" deliveries too, doesn't it?

Do you know I've been intending to send you birthday greetings since Sept. 9—for I really thought of it then. But every time I wrote you I had so much to say that just couldn't be left out. So now you're 22—and a doctor. Well, it won't be long before I can tell you how it feels to be 23, and here I am wondering if I should let my hair grow so as to look older.

Yes, internships have me worried, too. There are four girls in our class—the most who have ever graduated from our school. Last year they turned down one on the excuse that they hadn't enough room for women interns. And the other three girls have faculty connections.

I've written to Bellevue Hospital to satisfy my brother, but to get in one must take a competitive exam in New York in December. So that lets me out. No, I am not planning on a fellowship at Mayo's— but I'm surely hoping and praying for one. I'm really afraid to look forward to it, though. I probably haven't a chance. But at least I can say I knew you "when."

I finally heard from Mary. She had a wonderful trip to Mexico City and expects to go back to Rochester about the middle of October.

So "Harbor Lights" is your favorite now. Right now "Can I Forget You" is near the top of my list—with, I must admit, "Harbor Lights" and one or two others. However, "Harbor Lights" has a special niche now.

I see that the Corn Huskers won their game again this weekend. I'll admit they have a mighty good coach, but I suspect that the Tigers could make some corn fly. Do you agree?

I hope you gave Uncle Mac my love. He was quoted in our surgery lecture the other day, but not agreed with. I wonder if it was a misquote or a mistake on our professor's part. I know Dr. MacCarty ought to know about gastric carcinomas.

Well, I must study for a quiz I missed when on my OB call. Besides, you deserve at least no more writing after having to wade through all this. But don't you dare make your letters a bit shorter. They're too short as it is.

Love,
Alice

OMAHA

Thursday, October 14

My dearest Alice:

I could not eat my dinner fast enough so I could come up and answer your letter. It is a real pleasure to receive them. It seems that we are just talking to each other.

I wish that you could be at least a few miles closer and I could go to see you often. Oh, for a return of this summer, if only for a couple of weeks.

Dr. Rutledge, from the Clinic, has spent quite some time in Omaha and at the house here. In fact, I am finding out more about the Clinic daily. Do you know that they have a method of estimating the number of patients in a waiting room by determining the CO_2 combining power of the air in it?

This position at the Neb. Children's Home is given to only one student a year and it carries no salary. I have about 21 children there and they keep me busy with colds, injuries, etc. But I can make the 8-mile drive in no time now.

Did I tell you that I left Nellie at home and am now driving Nancy, my Studebaker? She does very well for her age (10 years). Nellie is in the Hospital undergoing some major surgery. We hope that her convalescence is brief and satisfactory.

We are having our annual Nu Sig pheasant hunt at Clarkson this weekend. Most of the actives go out, and we usually bring back a few pheasant and have a big alumni dinner here a week or so later. My mother plans to entertain all of the fellows for dinner Sunday, and you can bet that we will have kolaches.

We are having freezing weather here now. I can imagine the lovely weather that you are having.

Today as I was standing near the radio and listening to "Harbor Lights," I finally realized just why I like it. This may seem fantastic, but it does remind me of the light on the Clinic at Rochester and our meetings this summer—and then both of us leaving to be separated by miles and miles. May we meet again.

With love,
Joe

NEW ORLEANS
Tues. nite, Oct. 19

Dear Joe—

I had a perfect weekend, even if it did rain every minute of the time. I decided at the last minute Sat. to go home. It is nice to realize that your folks really appreciate you, especially when you've been away and can't stay long—Ha.

Earlier, I took all my collection of notes and papers from Mayo's to Ellanor Lockhart in the hospital, and she seems to be enjoying it. She started her internship in July and in Sept. discovered she had a minimal tuberculous lesion. The poor kid is taking it very well, though. Much better, I suppose, than I ever could. I surely enjoy talking about this summer to her. She wanted that course herself but was told it wasn't being offered the summer she applied.

Poor Nellie, be very good to her, won't you? I suppose Nancy is alright, but Nellie holds a special place in my heart.

And you really hunt pheasant. The only ones I've ever seen have either been stuffed or in a zoo, so you'll have to excuse my ignorance.

I see where Dr. Edwin G. Bannick et al. have an article in the latest Journal of the AMA. Did you meet him at Rochester? He is so nice, and doesn't it give you a thrill to have met some of these recognized authorities?

My dear, you have made "Harbor Lights" an unforgettable thrill for me. It does make me miss you terribly, but your letters help so much. And now I am getting silly. But may I echo your "May We Meet Again."

You should have heard what my mother said about your picture. I suppose you've learned to control your head size by now, but she said some mighty nice things, and she says you don't look exactly mentally deficient, either. I've learned that she is really a good judge of character—from times when we didn't agree so perfectly on our opinions of people as we do in this case.

I'll be looking forward to a letter soon.

My love—
Alice

OMAHA
Thursday, Oct. 28

Dear Alice:

A few minutes to spare before I go to the library, but I enjoy writing to you more. However, I cannot match stationery with you—and what a medical center you must have. I hope to see it someday. What a grand building.

I would give anything to go to Charity to intern but according to the Dean here, that is practically an impossibility. Consequently, I must be content with University Hospital here, if I can get in. What a worry this internship matter has turned out to be.

The freshmen at the house here are having quite a strenuous week—examinations in embryology and bacteriology. Gee, it would be quite a letdown to go back to that again, but I bet I could learn a lot now. In fact, I enjoy reviewing my pharmacology now, but I detested it during my sophomore year. Perhaps it was the instructor that I did not like.

My room seems to be the lounging place of everyone in the house so now I am having difficulty in writing. If this keeps up there will not be room to sit in here.

Have you seen the "Good Earth"? I know it is an old picture but it is late here. Didn't it portray in a typical way the way that many men treat their wives? Have you read the book by Pearl Buck? I divide some of my spare time between Irving & Poe this month.

And now, to the tune of Rudy Vallee singing "Goodnight Sweetheart," I must close.

Love,
Joe

New Orleans
Tues. Nite, Nov. 2

Dearest Joe—

I'm glad you like my stationery. I didn't realize the LSU medical school building was so impressive—but I assure you that, surrounded as it is by the old buildings of Charity and by the construction of the new Charity, it doesn't make nearly so nice a picture. However, I agree that you should come see it for yourself.

And I surely agree about the worry of internships. Our dean gave a very scorching talk about applying at a large number of places—just after I had received 4 very nice looking application blanks—and told us to get in our applications for Charity at once. But what worried me more, he offered me an internship in pathology. It was rather tempting, but I just can't see missing the chance for a year's general internship. Also, I understand that a general internship is required before one can get a fellowship at Mayo's, so that settled it. I just hope they'll take me here for I don't think I'll apply anywhere else.

So Nebraska is still in the lead. I'm as proud as if I went there myself. And I was so glad Notre Dame beat Minnesota. I don't know why except that Minnesota has been the big winner for so long. This seems to be a year of upsets.

I envy you your reading. How do you ever find time for Irving, Poe, and Pearl Buck? I must waste a lot of time because it seems I never have time to do anything except study and see a few shows. I think "The Life of Emile Zola" is one of the best ever. Have you seen it? I didn't get to see "Good Earth" but I read most of it—in magazine form. Paul Muni is a wonderful actor, isn't he?

I must stop as I have to study. We change medicine sections this week in addition to having a written in surgery, soooo—By the way, Shep Fields with his Rippling Rhythm is to be in New Orleans this Sat. nite. I can't imagine anything I'd enjoy more than dancing to his music with you. Of course, any other orchestra would do. Well, maybe—someday—

Love,
Alice

OMAHA
Sunday morning, Nov. 7
11:30

Dearest Alice:

I am a trifle sleepy this morning due to the fact that I got in at 5:30 a.m. from an OB and could not sleep any later than 10:00. About four more deliveries and I will be through. My roommate just got up and is ready to go to church so I will finish this later.

1:00

Just returned and my room is full of fellows reading the Sunday papers. Well, I hope they keep quiet for a short time at least.

We had our national Nu Sig secretary visit our chapter last Sunday, so the day was filled with banquets, speeches, and meetings. It was truly very inspiring to talk to a man who had been actively connected with the fraternity for 31 years. The more intimately that I am connected with NΣN, the more I am proud of the day that I pledged the fraternity. How is your sorority progressing? Just grand, I bet.

I plan to see the Dean in a final conference about my internship tomorrow. Neb. appoints Nov. 15th.

Imagine, we received an assignment of 32 pages in orthopedics last Friday. What a shock. I believe that our senior year is much easier than yours. We have not had any examinations yet, and it is rumored that they draw the final grades out of a hat in one course. However, I am not lucky in that respect.

Neb. has not been doing so well recently—quite a letdown. LSU certainly gave Mississippi a beating.

The "trucking" craze has hit Omaha—what a riot. I refuse to learn it, which may make me a dance outcast. However, I do not like dances here anyway. It is difficult to dance with someone else when I would much rather dance with you. In fact, even drinking a Coca-Cola together would be an unforgettable pleasure like it always was. Memories deeply treasured.

Now I have to put a dressing on a sprained ankle or the patient will be calling me.

Love,

Joe

NEW ORLEANS

Tues. Nite, Nov. 9

Dearest Joe—

The joke is on us. We thought that in finishing Medicine section, we would be preparing for 7 weeks of comparatively light work with OB, Gyn, and Newborn. But since my name is at the top of the alphabet, I'm having it piled on. Our Gyn department has the nicest way of giving us the history and some of the physical examination of a patient and expecting us to diagnose the case. The funny part is that there is always some question you need to have answered before you are sure of the diagnosis!

We were greatly honored this Saturday by a visit and talk by Journal of the American Medical Association editor Dr. Morris Fishbein. However, I personally wish he hadn't come. I heard him speak two years ago and was very favorably impressed. He is a remarkable orator and his lectures, while educational, are also interesting and just humorous enough. However, he spoiled that impression Saturday, for he picked out the female sex to insult and—well, he made every girl who listened to him furious. Not content with belittling our mental capacity, he informed the group that one only had to look around even in a medical class to see how women wasted money on cosmetics. Needless to say, it wasn't appreciated.

Seriously though, he gave us something to really worry about. He berated Charity Hospital in no uncertain terms. However, as long as I've known anything about it, Charity has been in a terribly crowded condition. Even before they tore down the old hospital building, there have been patients two in a bed or sleeping on the floor. So I can't understand the sudden commotion now when they really have an excuse for it. I surely hope he doesn't discredit the hospital. That would ruin my chance at a fellowship at Mayo's.

A pediatrics and gynecology case later

Don't you enjoy newborn service in Pediatrics? My only trouble is that I hate to see so many precious babies sent to orphan asylums. What will I do when I intern in that service! I suppose it's a good thing that there are so many that one couldn't possibly adopt them all.

Don't you think Nellie—or Nancy—would enjoy a little jaunt down to see the Sugar Bowl game, or Mardi Gras? I'd guarantee you a welcome.

What a volume, and I feel as if I could just keep on writing. Funny—I don't usually have that trouble! But I don't usually enjoy doing anything so much as I do when I do it with you. See what you get for being the nicest person I've met.

> Love,
> Alice

OMAHA

Friday, Nov. 12

Dearest Alice:

We are changing services this Saturday. I will have my schedule full with Gyn, OB, and Newborn. I have the same feeling about the little infants who have no place to live. In fact, one brutal mother stated that she does not care whether her child lives or not. That is not the motherly love that I know about.

Well, it is all over, I have my contract signed at the University. So now I will be in Omaha another year. We have a nice service—230 beds, 12 interns, 1 resident in Radiology, one in Pathology, and one in OB and Gyn. It involves a lot of responsibility, but we get to do a lot of surgery ourselves (such as appendices and groin hernia repair). But I am set on going to Mayo's in one year (if I can get in).

If I continue on my thesis on climate, I will cease believing in bacteria and blame all disease on the weather. Radical thought—perhaps due to Dr. MacCarty's influence.

Incidentally my roommate, A.C. Cimfel, received his acceptance from Dr. MacCarty last week for next summer's fellowship. I hope he is as fortunate as I was in meeting a girl such as you at the Clinic. Do you realize we have Uncle Mac to thank for our friendship?

"The Life of Emile Zola" certainly incited me to deep thought. It portrays that nothing can stop success if an individual believes in his ideas and strives even against overwhelming odds. Reviewing the life histories of several great men, we find that most of them were ridiculed at first, but their theories were later accepted, even if after their death. In other words, there is still much to be done in the field of medicine, and let us do our share—not for private and personal gain, but for the benefit of the profession and the multitude. I had better quit philosophizing or you may tear up this letter.

My opinion of Dr. Fishbein has certainly decreased enormously since I read your letter. How can such a man, in whom is entrusted such a great office, be so narrow-minded as to believe that women have no place in medicine? I thoroughly disagree with him. Although my experience with lady physicians is limited—namely, you and Dr. Stastny—I hold them in the highest esteem. And the crack about cosmetics—does he ever stop to figure how much money doctors waste on tobacco and liquor?

I cannot state for certain when I will come to visit you but it will be sometime—perhaps next spring. It would be most enjoyable, I know, and I appreciate the invitation.

Listening to the radio gives me the blues and makes me wish New Orleans was closer. "So Many Memories of You" and of "Whispers in the Dark" and then I get "That Old Feeling" about "The First Time I Saw You." I could go on like that forever.

Love,

Joe

NEW ORLEANS
Monday Nite, Nov. 15

Dearest Joe—

I've been dreading to see June come. It means the end of the care-freeness of school days and the beginning of true responsibility—but now, since it means the chance of a visit to the Sunny South for you, it is one of the shining landmarks to look forward to.

I wish you could enjoy the beautiful weather we've been having. Or is your Indian summer still with you? Just cool enough to be pleasant but not even requiring a light coat. And we still have some lovely flowers blooming. It's too bad winter has to come.

I'm sure you've heard the old saying about each person you meet bringing out some different response from you—and the advice to pick out someone who to you symbolizes the highest type of personality. For the first time I'm beginning to realize the truth of these statements. Heretofore I've usually soon been disappointed in my choice, but my friendship with you has proved increasingly inspiring, and I know my admiration has not been misplaced. So please continue your philosophizing.

We are really getting some neuro-psychiatry this year, and I find it particularly interesting. My new Social Service case is a neurotic. She has been an invalid for the past nine years but supposedly has nothing wrong. And she's only about 30 years of age! I believe cases like that deserve much more consideration than they are often given. After all, the physician's duty is not to cure and prevent death but to prolong a happier life—recognize Uncle Mac? And surely such a person must be one of the world's most unhappy creatures.

I wish I could be sure about my internship. I suppose we shan't find out for sure until around Christmas. I'll surely be in a fix if I get turned down here. Dot is applying for an internship in Radiology. She has been working with her brother Charles, taking his X-rays, and giving an occasional treatment, for the past two years.

I shall be wishing for a Nellie or Nancy tomorrow. The Hospital for Mental Disorders is quite a walk away from school. However, we ought to see some cases which will be well worth the trouble.

I must stop—I fear I write until I bore you. If so, any complaint will be appreciated. However, I'm not making any promises. When I start writing you I have to limit myself by the number of sheets or your punishment would be endless.

Love,
Alice

OMAHA
Thursday Noon, Nov. 18

My Dearest Alice:

I just received your letter and cannot answer it soon enough. You mention a complaint—the only one that I have is that your letters are not long enough. In fact, if they would be 50 pages long they would still be too short. They are so delightfully interesting I read and reread them.

We have had quite a sudden change in temperature and weather with about 3 inches of snow. It is about 15° above zero and that is much too cold—what will I do when it will be 20° below? Nancy will start to suffer now, this cold weather is very hard on her, but I hope that she will live through it. I just got through shoveling the snow off her.

5:30 p.m.

Just returned from a lecture on dietetics. We have to make out diabetic, obesity, nephritic and other diets, which is not so difficult, but today the dietitian made us eat some of the food which we prescribed, such as gravy made with mineral oil or 30 grams of butter with one meal. Yes, I pity the patients.

I finally got to see the slides from an autopsy that I did over a week ago on a case of encephalitis. Looking through a binocular reminded me so much of this summer, only you were not here to help me with the diagnosis.

Now I must dress for dinner.

10:30

What an evening—first a showing of a film by the Mead Johnson Company followed by three hours of Nu Sig committee meetings. The house committee meeting resulted in an agreement to elect an alumni committee and work through them. But the financial committee—what a mess. Imagine my predicament—two of my best friends are not able to pay their dues, and we have to act on suspending them. What an embarrassing situation. This office certainly is very time-consuming, but if it is to be done, it must be done right, and I will do it that way regardless of time.

You mention that our friendship is increasingly inspiring. I have never known anyone I have admired more than I admire you. Now, I must endeavor to live up to the high ideals that you know that I hold. I found a quotation in my files which I also try to follow— "Don't try to be an earthly saint with your eyes fixed upon a star— but try to be the kind of a fellow that your mother thinks you are."

It seems that our friendship deepens every time that I receive a letter from you. Oh, to live the summer over. Will we ever get to take our moonlight ride by horseback?

The sandman is calling but I almost dread going into the dormitory tonight—windows are never closed and it is snowing outdoors. Very invigorating, but we do not waste much time getting into bed. Someday, I fear, I will awaken under a blanket of snow.

I hope that you have a wonderful Thanksgiving. Will you please send the next letter to Clarkson? I shall be expecting it.

Love,
Joe

New Orleans

Mon. Nite, Nov. 22

Dearest Joe—

Probably when you get this, turkey will be occupying most of your mind. I hope you can manage to get the pulley bone and share a Thanksgiving wish with me.

The thermometer has been hovering between 30 and 40° for the past four days and is New Orleans complaining! I guess we just can't take it. We don't know how to cope with cold weather, and snow is such an oddity that it means a holiday for the school children.

I just got back from a meeting of the Orleans Parish Medical Society where a Dr. John B. Hawes from Boston spoke on the diagnosis of tuberculosis. He prefaced his remarks by saying that he hoped we wouldn't hold it against him because he was a Yankee. If he only knew how highly I esteem Yankees—at least some of them!

Our holidays begin the 24th, and although they last until the 29th, our biggest football game, LSU vs. Tulane, is played here on the 27th, so I expect the majority of us will be back for it.

I hate to close a letter to you. It's like stopping a conversation that I should never want to stop. My only consolation is that the sooner I get this letter off, the sooner I can hear from you. The best of Thanksgivings to a fellow whose mother must be thankful for such a son.

Love,

Alice

CLARKSON
Thanksgiving Day

My Dearest Alice:

Your letters came just in time to make this a perfect Thanksgiving Day. My thoughts of turkey were second to thoughts of you.

My sister, brother-in-law, nephew, and grandmother were at our home for the day and did I eat. We had everything, including strudel, kolaches, knedliky, and zali. Now I won't have to eat for weeks.

I never realized until today just how much I have to be thankful for—the grandest father and mother, a good education, an internship, no debts, health, and a lady friend in New Orleans who has been a great inspiration to me during the past few months. I suppose that you are spending your Thanksgiving with your parents, and I hope that you are as happy as I am.

It is quite a change to return to a town where you know everyone and they all know you. And they all ask, "How do you like school?" The young doctor (Clarkson's most eligible bachelor) has married a girl from Omaha, much to the disappointment of many of our home-town girls, some of whom had decided to take nurses training due to his influence.

But it is a grand town after all. We see people as they really are since they cannot put on a bright front to cover up a dark or shadowy interior as they do in the cities.

I spent a very enjoyable Saturday evening with Dr. Stastny last week. The more that I come in contact with her, the more I realize how great she is. She has been nationally recognized for her Red Cross work in Czechoslovakia and Greece after the war. She organized the first nurses training school in Prague. The conditions must have been horrible—some of the largest hospitals in Europe had no requirements whatsoever for their nursing staff. In fact, women who failed in every kind of occupation, even the lowest, were taken in as nurses. If anyone can succeed in raising such standards to those of the present, she should be admired. No, not another Florence Nightingale, but a worthy successor, and she has probably aided more people than most doctors in Omaha. And then Dr. Fishbein says that women have no place in medicine. As a criticism to that I am having Dr. Stastny come to the house and give a lecture on "Women in Medicine."

We had an alumnus over last Tuesday night, and he gave a lecture on medical ethics. The majority of his talk centered on the Hippocratic Oath, which he called the Constitution of Medicine. It is remarkable how much foresight that old man had 2,200 years ago.

We have a talk such as this every two weeks, and they prove of infinite value.

You should see my nephew —3 months old and weighs 16 pounds—yes, a little overweight but very active. I hope the pictures that I took of him come out.

And now, till we meet again—very soon I hope.

Love,
Joe

NEW ORLEANS
Mon. nite, Nov. 29

My Dearest Joe—

Well, we really have some week before us. Winning the football game gave us a holiday today, and the Southern Medical Convention gives us holidays thru Friday. All this following the Thanksgiving holidays is truly a treat. I shall be wishing you could be with me every minute of the time. Memories of Wednesday nite staff meetings will never be forgotten.

I had a most enjoyable Thanksgiving. The turkey was a huge one but didn't last long. My folks, strange as it may seem, always seem glad to see me. Seriously, it seems the more I'm away from home, the more I miss them—when I have time to miss anyone. My folks are getting rather old now, and I'm sorry I can't be with them more. It's a shame that one doesn't learn to really appreciate his folks until he leaves home. I hope someday I can make things a little easier for them—and have them with me, wherever that may be.

Your Dr. Stastny must indeed be a great woman and a great doctor. I was amazed to learn that women played such an active part in medicine during the World War. She and other pioneer women have given us a great inspiration—and a challenge to live up to. I hope I can someday be worthy of being called a "real doctor." She must be a personification of my meaning of that term, which to me is the ultimate of human goodness, kindness, and helpfulness. I'm beginning to understand your pride in her friendship.

Joe, you really made my heart skip a beat when you ended by saying you hoped we might meet again very soon. Isn't it a shame that miles have to be so long!

Love,
Alice

New Orleans
Monday p.m., Dec. 13

Dearest Joe—

We had our school dance Sat. nite, and I kept thinking how nice it had been this summer dancing with my favorite partner and not being surrounded with people who think that a dance means a drunken brawl. Every time I get so disgusted watching the way people act on such occasions, I think of you and am so thankful I know someone who realizes that good clean fun is best—and more enjoyable, I think. Gosh, don't I sound like a lecturing old maid aunt or something? Well, maybe I am, at that, but I'll still think of this summer as one of the most enjoyable times I have ever spent.

Dot has received notice of acceptance as an intern in Radiology, and Gretchen Vitter, another girl in our class, in Pathology. However, the general internships haven't been announced yet, so I'm still keeping my fingers crossed.

Eight members of our class are going to intern at Charity Hospital in Shreveport, three at Touro Hospital here in New Orleans, one is hoping for an internship at Los Angeles, California, and I think some of the class (northern Jews) are planning to go back East. We have quite a few of them in our school, and they're very good students. It seems they limit the number admitted to the eastern schools.

I sympathize with you in your attempt to stop smoking. I finally acceded to my mother's wishes and promised to stop smoking toward the end of the summer. So I haven't smoked a cigarette since the last of August. So it can be done, even though I'm greatly tempted when I see others enjoying it.

It seems I'm running out of paper, so perhaps I'd better stop—Till Monday, then.

My love,
Alice

OMAHA
Thursday, Dec. 16

My Dearest Alice:

We are having a Christmas party for the children from the Nebraska Children's Home at the house tomorrow night—with a Santa Claus and everything. I am certain that all of them should enjoy it. We feel that this may aid in enabling them to have a merry Christmas even though they have no home.

I had some nice experience at the Home this Tuesday. One of the 13 year old boys broke both bones in the lower one-fifth of the forearm while sleigh riding. It happened rather late in the day, and I could not get him into the Uni, so I had to set it there. He wants to be a G-man, so while he was "shooting gangsters" I did the manipulation. A peach box furnished the splints. This happens to be the first arm that I ever set, and was I surprised when the X-ray showed the bones in place. Wasn't I fortunate that they slipped into place? Accidents do happen and luck was with me.

Monday it started raining and soon it turned into sleet, thereby coating everything with ice. Imagine how difficult it would be to drive on a skating rink—that is just the way the streets of Omaha were. Brakes are of no advantage on a car. In fact, they tend to make a sled out of it —and where you stop, nobody knows. From now on until March, the only safe way to drive is with chains, and all we hear is their continuous clanging against icy pavement and occasionally the roar of an automobile motor whose owner decided to do without them and the wheels spin without moving the car.

But the winter weather does have its beauty. It is very inspiring to look outdoors after a heavy snowstorm and see the boughs of the fir trees bending down with their overburden of snow, the automobiles breaking new trails in heretofore untred places (almost a pioneering spirit)—and the peace and quiet that exists, as if the entire vicinity had been covered with a blanket of good will and beauty. However, you can make up your own mind about winter when you get to Rochester. It gets 30° below there—almost time for red flannels. Sometimes I wish that I had a pair when I go on an outcall miles north.

We have the same attitude about dances and "drunken brawls." I cannot see the logic of anyone getting inebriated and not being conscious of their acts. And the next morning, after they have taken all the Acetyl salicylic acid in the house and with ice caps on their heads, they say, "Gee, I had a swell time." We will both be old-fashioned and drink our Coca-Colas, and occasionally a little beer.

I must say that it is very rare to see a girl with that attitude, and I am proud that I have met her. And I admire anyone who quits smoking, particularly because her mother wishes her to do so.

I completed my OB and Gyn dispensary today and now I wonder what comes next, perhaps laboratory.

Later

Had another call to the home—a little girl bumped her head, and I hope it is not a skull fracture.

I wish that you could be here to help us entertain the children tomorrow, but more just so I could see you again.

May I wish you a very joyous Christmas and a happy and successful New Year filled with gratification of all of your desires.

I'll be in Clarkson for 2 weeks.

Love,

Joe

ALEXANDRIA

U.S.V.A.

Monday, Dec. 20

Dearest Joe—

It was such a joy to get your cards and letter this morning. Dad had to call me to the table—I had forgotten about dinner.

Your cards are so nice and mean so much more than an ordinary card. Mr. Dennis is a real fellow, isn't he? I'll bet he's the center of attraction this week, and justly so. There's nothing that makes for a true Christmas more than a baby to enjoy it with.

I'm so proud of you. That must have been a job to set a small boy's leg like that. It sounds as if you didn't even have an anesthetic! I'll hand it to you. And there's a lot more than luck to the setting of bones. You're certainly to be congratulated.

I've been running around this week without any wrap on at all. The sun is warm and nice—even an occasional flower is in bloom. Dad got some holly and mistletoe from the woods yesterday, and they're so pretty—just loaded with berries. It's very nice but hardly seems like Christmas. I can remember two Christmas seasons when we had enough snow to call it a white Christmas, but even then it was stretching the point somewhat. However, we are so unprepared for cold weather here that we'd probably freeze before we know it if it did get truly cold. Dad has had his toes frostbitten and declares he'd never go north again—

That is, until we start talking about Mayo's. Then he tells me that he wouldn't mind spending the summers in Minnesota. I've been wondering if I should be considering going so far away from them for so long a time. Dad is to be retired in a couple of years, and I don't know what they are going to do with themselves. Dad says he's going to catch up on his fishing and not work, but I know that won't last.

I'm surely glad, though, that they both seem to want me to go to Mayo's if I get the opportunity.

I'm sure you are having a very full and happy vacation. I hope Santa is kind and Christmas a most joyful time. Its spirit is a wonderful thing and certainly puts us in a fine mood to begin our New Year, which I'm sure will be filled with worthy accomplishments and deserved commendations for you.

Love,
Alice

"THE KAHLER"
ROCHESTER, MINN.

Wed. evening, Dec. 22
9:45

My Dearest Alice:

How I miss you tonight—more than I ever have, which is quite a lot.

I imagine that my presence in Rochester demands an explanation. Mrs. Sedlak, my sister's mother-in-law, has been ill with some gastro-intestinal distress (perhaps malignancy or diverticulosis) for the past month, so we came to Mayo's this morning. She is in Dr. Edgar Allen's clinic. I expect to go back home tomorrow.

Something is lacking in Rochester—you. I was at the staff meeting tonight and, gee, it felt tough to sit alone.

Memories of this summer are all around me. Nothing much has changed in the town except that it is awfully cold here, even for me. But we still can use the tunnels.

Met Dr. Bargen, and he invited me to his clinic at Dr. MacCarty's tomorrow. I hope they have a good fight. I must see Uncle Mac tomorrow and my friend Dr. Rutledge.

Alice, the more that I am here the more I am agreed that we should come up for fellowships. And we must work hard for them, starting now.

Went to the apartment at noon, and truthfully I was disappointed when I did not see your smiling face at the door. Mary almost fainted. Her parents are here. Had dinner there tonight and, gee, I wish you had been there.

Mary is very enthused about her work as head of the welfare department's Civic League—had a radio program tonight soliciting gifts for the needy—and so far she has been very successful. She is certainly happy. Mr. & Mrs. Lomasney are very nice people. Isn't Mary a picture of her mother?

I have been at home only 2 days but will spend 10 days there after I return. I must go to get your letter tomorrow.

Again may I wish you a most happy Christmas and a successful New Year. Now I will watch the "Harbor Light" on my way to my room. Till we meet again.

All my love,
Joe

CLARKSON
Saturday, Dec. 25
1:25 a.m.

My dearest Alice:

We just returned from Midnight Mass, which was a most beautiful service. Now, by the light of the fire and Christmas candles, I must write to you.

Thank you billions for the wonderful photo you sent me. It is just what I have wanted for the past 5 months. It looks so lifelike, and anytime I expect you to step out of the frame and speak to me—if you only could.

I have had a nice Christmas. The spirit of giving is something that we should never lose.

Sleet started to fall this morning, and now everything is covered with a fine, glistening layer of ice. The coated branches reflect the light like so many diamonds in the trees. More work for Argus tomorrow.

I returned from Rochester at noon after spending an awful night on the train—17 hours to make a trip that Nancy or Nellie could make in 10. Mrs. Sedlak stayed there—it is probably diverticulosis.

I went to Uncle Mac's laboratory Thursday, but he was gone for the day. Many of the fellows are new, and two Chinese woman physicians are there too. Of course, all I heard was about the Sino-Jap War. Gee, but the lab looked empty without you—I expected you to walk out of one of the rooms any minute.

Why cannot we turn time back 5 months?

One classroom was changed into a party room with a Christmas tree, fireplace, etc., and the pathology fellows and assistants had a party at 11 with coffee, sandwiches & cake, so of course I got to stay.

Nothing has changed at the Clinic or St. Marys except for Christmas decorations. The Chapel at the Hospital is beautiful now.

Surgery is the same—Dr. Adson still talks constantly.

Attended Dr. Bargen's ward round. Since Dr. MacCarty was gone there was no clinic.

And Thursday afternoon it was time for me to visit Dr. Wilder's diabetic clinic, but he does not conduct them anymore. Met him in the library & he remembered Dr. Baker from New Orleans.

And Friday, time for Dr. Hench's ward round—but I was uncomfortably riding a train at that time.

I was very fortunate in being able to ride the same train as Dr. Allen, head of one of the departments of medicine and a Neb. graduate. He is a very young man and very brilliant.

Met Dr. Alice Grace Hildebrand—a Neb. grad of 1936 and now a fellow at the Clinic. She is in medicine and stated that there are 17 women fellows there. Of course, I tried to find out all about it for you. She made a personal application and started last July 1st.

But Rochester seemed empty without you—so the next best thing was to visit with Mary and hear her talk of you. She wants us to come up next summer.

I spent several hours in the library working on my thesis. Yes, I was quite busy during my 2-day stay there.

I imagine that you are having a very enjoyable Christmas at home. Too bad that your brother & sister cannot come. My grandmother is staying with us this winter. She is 78 and we do not want her to live alone, and we enjoy having her with us. I never saw anyone that old who reads as much as she does.

I hope that you forgive my awful scribbling, but I did have only 2 hours sleep on that awful train last night, and here it is 2 a.m. again.

I'm just crazy about your picture. Now the fellows at the house can see a picture of the girl I have been talking about ever since school started. And my parents think it is grand. Thank you again. Until Thursday.

Love,
Joe

ALEXANDRIA
Mon. nite, December 27

Dearest Joe—

I have really had a red letter day. Two letters and my beautiful gift, all on the same day. That vanity compact is the beautifullest thing I've ever seen, it really is. At first glance I realized that. Then I saw the NΣN crest and it meant much, much more, but when I finally caught my breath enough to look under it—well, you can imagine my surprise and delight. Mother said, "My, isn't he fine looking," and I was almost speechless but managed to agree with her. I wish I could just halfway tell you how proud I am of it.

I'll have to admit frankly that your visit to Rochester made me quite envious—of Mary or of anyone who got to see you—and so lonesome. It recalled this summer and all its good times so vividly, and it seemed as if I should be able to walk over to Mary's as of yore and see you all. But those old 1,100 miles are still there, it seems. I'm certainly looking forward to the day when I can just snap on some wings and fly wherever I want to go—some daydream—but I believe we'll do it just the same.

I know Mary must have had the best Christmas ever. She is so closely attached to her family, and with her job her joy must have been complete. I'll bet Mr. Lomasney told you some tales. When they lived in Louisiana, he used to keep Mary and me in laughter.

It's tragic to see the holidays slipping by so fast, but in a way I'm getting ready to get back to work already. It's hard work, this doing nothing—especially with no one to do it with.

Of course that isn't quite true, but Mother is kept at home almost constantly with my aunt, and it's when we get out together that we rejoice. My uncle Charlie Baker is also with us now. He is crippled— the result of a cerebral hemorrhage last year—and the inactivity is so hard on him.

Oh, did I tell you I got my internship all right? They took 34 from our class of 58, plus 25 Tulane students and 23 from other schools. Lyne Gamble from Vanderbilt—remember him?—was accepted. I'm wondering if he'll take it. I agree perfectly that we should get Mayo fellowships and am certainly hoping I can get in. There's no question about your success, and I'm going to do my best. I'm so proud that Dr. Wilder remembered me, and that Dr. Holoubek thought enough of me to mention me—and I do think they need more women fellows, don't you?

Gosh, there's so much I'd like to tell and ask you. And thanks for thinking of me Christmas night. The thought was mutual.

Mother and Dad asked me to thank you for the card. It was lovely (after asking me who J. E. Holoubek could possibly be. Do they like to kid me!) and they really appreciate it.

Best wishes to you and all your family for the best year ever.

My love—
Alice

'Your voice sounded so nice'

January–June 1938

Monday, Jan. 3

Dearest Joe—

I doubt if you will be able to read a word of this. I know I can't. I had my eyes examined today, since Monday afternoon is the only one we get off—and with my dilated pupils I can't even see what I'm writing. But if I didn't get to write my Mon. nite letter I would be too disappointed, for I don't want to chance yours being late.

Dr. H.F. Brewster, the ophthalmologist who examined my eyes and who is an instructor at LSU, told me something funny. He said I had never looked like the type of girl who would study medicine. I wonder what type of girl is supposed to study medicine. Then he added that I looked as if I were the type who wouldn't be completely happy until married and a mother of six. I hardly knew what to say but managed to agree when he said medicine needn't necessarily prevent that. Isn't it funny how people who are practical strangers become interested in one's affairs?

Your Dennis is a most intelligent and healthy looking youngster, and he looks as if he would enjoy being pals. I've been wishing I could see a picture of his mother. She must be a very pretty and lovable girl, to be who she is.

Oh, and do I feel proud showing off my vanity. Everyone who sees it agrees that it is the loveliest one they've ever seen, and that picture idea is a new one to us here. And am I proud of that NΣN crest—and just think, the president of the chapter gave it to me.

You should see George, the cute little boy we have on pediatrics ward. He has eyelashes as long as Marlene Dietrich's (even in the movies), and when he came in had a tummy full of hard balls. The diagnosis was much debated, but one of the students solved it when he found a roundworm crawling on the floor—some fun, eh!

Gee, I'd better not make you struggle through any more of this. I'll bet it's illegible. I'll try to write extra nice next time if you'll forgive this. Thanks so much for the pictures. I love to get them.

Love,
Same ole me

OMAHA
Wednesday, Jan. 5

Dearest Alice:

I just reviewed all of my surgery notes but I cannot say that I learned very much. Imagine, the faculty has the nerve to demand that the seniors take semester examinations this year. That is almost unprecedented.

This month I have the fullest schedule that I have ever had in medical school—8–5 Mon & Tue, 8–4 Wed-Fri and 9–3 Sat—with Urology, Orthopedics, Adult Heart, Dermatology & Syphilology, Neurology, and Allergy and TB as my dispensary services. Consequently, my thesis will not be completed this month.

The more that I read in medicine the more I agree with Dr. MacCarty about the chaos and lack of organization existing. One physician grades reflexes as 1+, 2+, 3+ and 4+ and it does not mean anything to the next man. We are given 3 different classifications for burns, 8 for nephritis. And, to top it off, we are taught the metric system and diligently learn it, and now we find that practically all staff men use the Apothecary system. And the nurses in the hospital never heard of cubic centimeters, grams, etc. Nevertheless, I like the metric and I expect to use it even though I have to unite them both.

Just received an outcall—the patient, 3 months old, has been vomiting all day. Now I have one case 51 blocks north and an OB 61 blocks south. Good old Nancy, I hope she holds together.

I will send more pictures whenever I get them finished.

I am surely proud of your portrait, and everyone in the house said, "Why not have her come to Neb. to school." Why not?

Love,

Joe

New Orleans

Mon. nite, Jan. 10

Dearest Joe—

Another Monday—and a walk home through the rain today at noon so I could get your letter sooner. Sir Aldo Castellani lectured to us this afternoon, keeping us from getting our usual afternoon off. Perhaps that is one reason why we were disappointed in him. So far, his lectures on tropical medicine have been informal and have held little new information. Last year, we heard him tell of his campaign of preventative medicine that he used during the Ethiopian war. And, I assure you, it was much more interesting than his review of pellagra. I understand he delivers 10 lectures to us during the year, for which he is paid $10,000. Not bad pay for ten hours, eh?

Your school hours sound terrific. Ours are never over 9–5 on weekdays and 9–1 on Saturdays. And occasionally, in our last two years, we get a few hours off. Our senior year is divided into 4 sections. We're in one of the easiest ones now—Pediatrics, Tropical

Medicine, and Neuro-Psychiatry. But in two weeks that will be over and we start Surgery. We all dread it although we enjoy it. With it we have Urology and Orthopedics. Of course, weekly medicine and surgery lecture and clinical pathological conferences continue throughout the year. And every Saturday we have "day clinic"— Surgery diagnostic clinic, where our chief, Dr. Urban Maes, gets to leisurely elaborate on various and sundry surgical cases. I really enjoy the hour. His characterization of a country doctor—smelling of antiseptic, with a thermometer in his mouth, and with an interesting case to report—is rather amusing, but he admits he wasn't a success as one and therefore was forced into city practice.

Ellanor Lockhart, the intern who contracted tuberculosis, is up again and doing part time OB duty. I'm still rather worried about her for her X-ray pictures have shown only a stationary lesion—no improvement—and she still has slight daily temperature. However, I know she's being very carefully watched.

Poor old Happy, my father's car, had a mishap—and on New Year's Day, too. I surely hope it's not a bad omen. I got him in the middle of the highway and killed the engine—and couldn't start him. A neighbor found the trouble but we had to ask for professional help. His locomotor and gastro-intestinal tract became disconnected.

I surely agree with you about confusing classifications in Medicine. Thank goodness, our medicine and clinical path departments got together and agreed on one classification which would be used here, so that's a great help.

Oh, you remember George, with his pet worms. Well, we found him on the contagious ward the other day with a beautiful case of chicken pox—which, according to the incubation period, he must have contracted while in the hospital.

I'm anxious to see the new pictures. So, until next Monday—

Love,
Alice

OMAHA
Monday, Jan. 10
11:15

Dearest Alice:

We have another comparatively warm day—only 32° above as compared to near zero last Friday to Sunday. Typical Nebraska weather, warm one day and cold the next.

Incidentally, I had a home delivery last Friday night. The patient lived near the So. Omaha stock yards. We were called at 11 p.m. and she delivered at 2 a.m. The house was heated by an old wood-burning stove. No running water. But a live baby boy was delivered.

We have to call a staff man and inform him when we are out on a case, and the nearest phone was at a fire station several blocks away. I decided to walk instead of taking Nancy, and did I freeze.

Now I have another patient, 18 years old, living on 16th and Dodge Street in an alley apartment. This is practically downtown so I do not expect too much trouble. She is due the 22nd of January. It is a crime that some of these girls bear children at such an immature age.

I received a letter from Dr. Allen from Mayo's today, and the final diagnosis on Mrs. Sedlak was bilateral hydronephrosis, which proves that conclusions should be reached only after an exhaustive examination and not a snap diagnosis like was made by her local physician.

Love,
Joe

OMAHA

Tuesday evening, Jan. 18

My Dearest Alice:

The Dean called me into his office last week. After a few uncomfortably long few minutes, during which I wondered just what he wanted, he stated that he found some new references for me for my thesis—journals from 1868 on. I started to write on the history of spas, this developed into history of climatotherapy—and now it will be climatology in all of its aspects.

We had a four-inch snow today—the heaviest of the season—and I took some very nice photographs. The campus looks beautiful—flower beds, drives, and terrace covered with soft fluffy snow. Would you enjoy sleigh riding? I would with you.

I should study for examinations, but this is so much more fun. We all applauded our medical jurisprudence instructor when he said, "It won't do you any good if I give you an examination, it won't help me, and the University will not profit—so why have one?" I wish more instructors would be like him.

I am listening to "You're a Sweetheart."

Love,

Joe

NEW ORLEANS
Sun. Nite, Jan. 23

Dearest Joe—

I just got back from a long, rainy bus ride from home—but a most enjoyable weekend. My Uncle Charlie had seemed unusually anxious to see me, so my folks wired me to come home. He is suffering almost continuously from vertigo, and although I can do nothing more than is being done for him, he seems to like to talk everything over with me. He has been my imaginary "Uncle Bim" (from "The Gumps") ever since I can remember, and to see him so helpless now is almost heart-breaking. But he is still young in spirit and enjoys nothing more than pulling a joke on someone. And he has such big plans for the future. I hope that, by some miracle, he will be able to carry them out.

We change sections this week, and our hardest section—surgery—begins.

Mother asked me about you Sat. nite, and I tried again to express to her my ideas of your fine, clean character, idealism, and natural gift of a charming personality. Then the subject turned to when I might possibly see you again. I said, "Oh, this June, I hope," and the thought was so pleasant that I carried it into my dreams. And everyone asked me why the "so happy" expression I was wearing around this morning.

Mon Nite

We started surgery with a bang! I had two cases assigned this morning, which I must have completely worked up by tomorrow at nine o'clock. And I'm probably the next one up for a case tomorrow. To make it worse, one of my patients had to pick today to be operated on. Our heartfelt thanks went out to our Path prof, who didn't believe in starting off without a week in which to catch our breath, and let us out of that class. Tomorrow the five in my section are on call for the Emergency room from 3–10 p.m., with cases being assigned right along. It's funny how we used to think we were abused when we got three medicine cases in one week. Well, at least, it will only last 7 weeks—and it's really most enjoyable work when one has time to catch his breath.

Goodness, it's 'most 9 o'clock and I haven't started writing my histories yet, so I suppose I'll have to stop this enjoyment and get to work. If you don't mind patchwork letters, I'm going to try to add a bit more before this goes out.

Tues a.m.

One of our new profs must be a newcomer in the Surgery Department, for he let us out a half hour early. I don't suppose it will happen again, but I'm glad it happened this morning.

Last night it was rather warm, and I got my first mosquito bite of the year. The wind from some nearby storm hit us, and it's rather cool today.

I've just discovered I'm assigned to diabetic clinic today and will miss my obstetric lecture. It's 'most time for the bell—in fact, there it is.

Until next week—

Love,
Alice

OMAHA
Thursday, Jan. 27

My Dearest Alice:

I was never so glad to see Thursday come—I needed some consolation and I can only get it from your letters. They are so inspiring, so interesting, but they always make me realize just how much I am missing by being unable to see you, talk to you, and to enjoy your companionship. It is true that we cannot have everything in life, but it seems that I am missing one of the best things.

Yes, the past two weeks have been quite a nightmare to all of us. After constant study and cramming, everyone became so irritable, but now it is all over and we hope that we all passed. Now only one more series of examinations next spring, which includes a three-hour comprehensive, and the state board on June 7th.

But after June 7th I hope that I will go south. Yes, I am making plans—oh, we could have so much fun, and I do not care if there would be a billion mosquitoes, just as long as you would be there. My father and mother are planning a trip through Oklahoma, Texas, Mexico, and La. Gee, I hope this materializes. Let us just hope and wait—4 ½ more months.

Our new semester starts Monday. For the next eight weeks I will be on University Outcall and will not have dispensary. Time to work on my thesis. During the second 8 weeks I will be on dispensary again with Lab, Oto-Rhino-Laryngology, and Pediatrics.

I am still waiting for my OB to deliver—one week overdue already—and I almost hesitate to go to bed tonight. Had quite an experience the other day when I called there and her twin sister came to the door—no, she wasn't pregnant. Embarrassing situation.

We have not received our intern instructions yet, but from what I hear we get no time off except when we sign out to the other interns. Each man has one ward and the work must be done there. We do our own lab work. And we get two weeks vacation.

Now all of the fellows have gathered in my room—post-mortems on the exams. One of the juniors has a make-up in surgery tomorrow. He does not seem too worried.

Nancy was in the hospital again today. A valve spring was broken and it interfered with the usual rhythm of knocks and bangs, so it had to be fixed.

I have visions of spending most of tonight on my OB, and I should get a few hours sleep now. In the meantime, I'll dream of you.

Love,

Joe

New Orleans

Thurs. Nite, Jan. 27

Dearest Joe—

We had several interesting cases on emergency service—a filling station attendant who was held up, robbed, and shot through the arm; a woman who was hit by a streetcar, causing a fracture of the hip; a Negro whom someone must have taken for a loaf of bread from the way he was sliced up, etc.

Today Dr. Arthur Myers, recently elected President of the National Tuberculosis Association, talked to us. His lecture, combined with some very interesting slides, made everyone present want to rush out for a tuberculin test. He attaches much more importance to this test as administered to adults than we were led to believe it had. He advocates it as a part of the routine physical examination of all public school and college students and teachers. I had thought that it was so commonly positive in adults that its only diagnostic value was in children. However, it seems I am wrong.

Sleigh riding sounds as the greatest of fun to me. Bernes Larson, the dietitian at Hotel Dieu Hospital here, has been describing the wonderful times she had at school on sleigh rides. She is from South Dakota but went to school in Minneapolis. We have so much fun talking about Minnesota. She says she gets lonesome for snow and all that goes with it, but I think she really enjoys the South.

Surgery, as usual, is calling. However, it isn't so important that I can't put it off for a while—just long enough to write to you. Cole Porter melodies on the radio—I do enjoy them. Songs give you so many pleasant memories and dreams. How dull living would be without them. I believe this past year has been about the happiest of all—and so many priceless memories result from 6 weeks of knowing you.

> Love,
> Alice

Oмана
Monday, Jan. 31

My Dearest Alice:

What a pleasure to relax and write to you after such a day like today—outcall, new services and, above all, Nancy went out for a count of ten. This time it is the clutch, last week, the valves. A constant source of worry—but where would I be without Nancy? When I recall the hours we spent ploughing mud, breaking trails through snow banks, and the times we took eight men to school when it was 20° below—a great pal, but not young anymore. Practically human—into the stage of senility—with complications ensuing. But we hope that the degeneration is not so great that a minor surgical procedure will not remedy it.

Finally I had my OB. After waiting here for two weeks I had hoped that she would not deliver until Sunday. The reason— "The Buccaneer" was here Sat. night for a Midwest preview. My roommate and I went, and just as Jean Lafitte discovered that his men had burned the Corinthian, my patient called me. 7 1/4 pound girl—and everything went fine even though it was zero outside.

Now I have to wait until next Thursday to see the show when it returns here. The part of it that I saw was very interesting—and I only hope that I can visit some of the scenes with you someday.

We had another cold spell last Saturday—and it finally got down to -8° this morning. A trifle cool. I hope that this is not a repetition of the three weeks of continuous below-zero weather that we had two years ago. Snow without such extreme cold is grand, but we get our climatic stimulation here—now, I am back to my thesis again.

I spent a very enjoyable evening at Dr. Stastny's last Friday. One of her friends, who had just returned from 9 months in the Orient, kept us busy all evening listening to her stories.

Incidentally, we are having Dr. Stastny over for dinner next week. Her subject of discussion will be European medicine, and her 16 trips to Europe should qualify her very well.

I have not been home for over a month but, with Nancy willing, I may go in two weeks.

Until Thursday.

Love,
Joe

New Orleans
Tues a.m., Feb. 1

Dearest Joe—

Greetings on this fine brrry morning—or do you listen to the
Breakfast Club? Anyway it's a fine morning here in New Orleans,
and so cold my nose is the color of a nice pickled beet!

I've been so excited since I read of your plans for June. It's all I
can do to keep my feet on the ground! Just imagine, to see and be
with you again, after all these months of remembering and dreaming and wishing. And how lovely that your father and mother are
going to have such a grand trip. I've been so anxious to meet them.
I'm sure it would be impossible not to think them the grandest
people ever. I surely hope they'll like Louisiana. Are you going to
get to make the complete trip with them?

Tell Nancy that I'm so anxious to meet her that she must keep her
good health 'til after this summer, at any rate. How is my old friend
Nellie? She'll always have a warm place in my heart.

Bernes Larson and I had quite a discussion the other day. We
decided the boys, as a whole, had cleaner minds up North than
down here. I suppose I have no right to judge, according to Dr.
MacCarty's principles, as I don't know many northerners, but if they
are all similar to the ones I know, there can be no doubt about it.

I was just telling my friends last nite that those six weeks this past
summer have meant more to me than most anything I can think
of. And when I think of how I almost didn't write Dr. MacCarty
because I was so sure I wouldn't get to go, and about how I wrote to
go the summer before, but he advised me to wait 'til the memorable
summer of 1937. Oh gee, it makes me thank my lucky stars.

I shall be eagerly awaiting a letter.

Love,
Alice

OMAHA

Friday, Feb. 4

My Dearest Alice:

I've lost all of my faith in cold vaccines. Today I have the biggest cold that I have had for years and, of course, I am using every remedy that I know—force fluids, acetyl sal, carbolfuchsin, Eucalyptus ointment, rest, Benzedrine Inhaler, etc., but seemingly to no avail. But with only two classes to skip tomorrow, I should be OK by Monday.

This is the unhealthiest weather that we have had for ages, oscillating from below zero to 60 above—in two days.

I had to see "The Buccaneer" yesterday afternoon before I decided to treat my cold, and this time I got to see the entire show without interruption. Will we ever have the opportunity to row through the same beautiful views that Lafitte did after the priests were captured—but, of course, we will not be trying to escape as they were. Now, more than ever, I want to go to New Orleans. How much of that story is actually true? You must tell me all about it sometime. If summer would only come soon.

But I am afraid that Nancy will not make the trip. I have not seen Nellie for five weeks, but she seems to be in good health.

We are starting a course in tropical medicine given by Dr. Claude Mason, who spent 19 years in the tropics. Many of his stories seem incredible. If we believe only one-half of them, they still seem impossible. But we fail to realize many things that take place in countries that we have not visited. Someone made a statement, "The world is a book, and he who stays at home reads but one page." I want to go south.

My OB patient is getting along nicely. The Visiting Nurses' Association takes care of the patient free of charge.

Our grades are not out yet—the office takes about a month before they send them out—but we have not heard any reports to the contrary, so perhaps we passed.

I had an argument with one of the fellows about "absence makes the heart grow fonder." I maintained that it did. Almost six and one-half months since I saw you—it seems like years—and I get more anxious everyday. Six weeks together last summer—memories that will last for a lifetime. Yes, how fortunate that we went last year—and if I had not pledged NΣN, I would never have heard of the summer course. Certain factors have a very great influence upon our lives and destinies. Until Monday.

Love,
Joe

OMAHA
Monday, Feb. 7

My Dearest Alice:

Another night at the library and my books came from the Mayo library. One, W.F. Peterson's "The Patient and the Weather," is in four parts and must contain thousands of pages. Now to make more maps and charts. A few more weeks and I should have the thesis completed but, as I told the Dean today, it is only a start and may develop into some investigative work eventually.

We had some excitement here at noon today. About the time that we sat down to lunch, the cook came running out of the kitchen and screamed that a fire had started there. Realizing it was out of control, we called the fire department and calmly sat down to finish our lunch while smoke rolled out of the kitchen and fire sirens shrieked. By the time we were ready for our dessert, the fire was out and smoke cleared—and quite a crowd of spectators had gathered. No damage done.

Nancy is running, on occasion. Very interesting case, her illness. Diagnosis—malfunction of the gears. Etiology—old age. Pathology—a few teeth broken out of the fly-wheel.

I plan to see "King Richard II" here Wednesday night. It is rare that we get to witness such a good production here.

I read A.J. Cronin's "The Citadel" this weekend. It seems that the character Dr. Manson played a Dr. Jekyll & Mr. Hyde existence. I admired him starting out in the mining town, fighting against great obstacles in Aberdeen, obtaining his M.D., always true to his wife and living up to the ideals that he had set for himself. But it was a bitter disappointment to see him become a society doctor, a "pill peddler," and acquire a lust for money. But the ideals must have been strong because he finally gave up everything for them. Look what he could have done if he had maintained them throughout. Above all, let us always stick to our ideals no matter how much criticism we must suffer. Too many doctors are very enthusiastic but soon crumble and join the crowd of mediocre men. But why follow the crowd? I don't crave money. All I ask is a place to practice medicine the way that I want to do it. Twenty years from now I expect to have the same attitude.

Will you be at Galvez 2-753 at 8 p.m. Feb. 14th? I would enjoy talking to you on St. Valentine's Day.

Love,

Joe

OMAHA
Thursday, Feb. 10
11:40 p.m.

My Dearest Alice:

I just took Dr. Stastny home. We had a delightful time here listening to her experiences in Czechoslovakia, Greece, and France. I am enclosing a bit of information that I used in introducing her for the after-dinner speech. Incidentally, one of the main reasons I invited Dr. Stastny over for dinner and for a talk is to convert the fellows to my method of thinking—that women play a very important part in medicine. Yes, we get into some heated arguments about that topic. Perhaps if they would all be as fortunate as I am in knowing you, they would agree with me.

We are certainly busy on outcall. Four new cases today added to the list—empyema, rheumatic fever, chicken pox, and neurosis following shell shock. Visiting the patients is not half as hard as finding the homes. Some live in basements, others in alleys, etc. And we did get a breath of fresh air when we got out into the country to see a case of chicken pox.

I am starting to file all of my reading material as well as index all of the articles I read in connection with medicine. It is a lot of work, but someday I hope to have a workable file and index. And, incidentally, I am starting a record of my mistakes—yes, there are a lot of them, but there will never be the same ones made twice.

And now four blood smears on my desk—must be counted before afternoon calls tomorrow. Would not it be grand if you and I could make our calls together? And after that—the theatre, dance, etc.

I'll be so anxious to see you this summer. And you must meet my parents. Let's not plan too much because something could happen. But I still want to see the Gulf Coast, sail on the ocean, and talk to you. Yes, I am planning and dreaming.

I saw Maurice Evans in "King Richard II" last night and enjoyed it very much. We are certainly getting initiated into the life of an M.D. now. I had a call just before I went to the play, and the only drug that worked was morphine (given, of course, by permission of a staff man).

I had planned to go home this weekend, but I must read my books and finish my reference work on the thesis.

Until Monday—when I expect to talk to you.

Love,

Joe

New Orleans

Fri. Morning, Feb. 11

Dearest Joe—

I've been so excited since I got your letter. To get to talk to you Mon. nite! You bet I'll be there. I'm so anxious to hear your voice.

I'll have to hand it to you and your fraternity brothers. You certainly should make good physicians. After hearing about how you ate your dinner right on through the fire in the kitchen, you must be the personification of "Aequanimitas," that imperturbability of which Dr. William Osler writes. If it were any other group of people, I might blame it on normal physiological grounds of hunger, but since you are embryo physicians, I'm sure it's your natural and acquired phlegm.

We have been asked to join the National Association of Medical Women. I don't understand exactly what the purpose is, and I wonder if it is advisable. I think it nice for there to be frequent association among medical women, but I don't think it advisable for them to try to segregate themselves too much from medical men. After all, the purpose of all is the same. We are probably excluded from some of the men's associations, and this is understandable in some instances. But I don't believe too marked attention should be paid to the difference in sex.

Of course, I'm probably wrong. I had my first disagreeable experience with a patient yesterday. A race track groom, alleged dope addict, decided I couldn't be a good doctor, that I was an "awful woman" to ask him such questions as is necessary to obtain a history. Well, he succeeded in making me so angry that I could hardly make myself examine him. He was very uncooperative. Well, I'm just hoping now that he deserts—and the sooner the better. I don't think he belongs on a surgery ward anyway.

At last, all the members of our class have obtained internships. And, from what we have heard about the new hospital, there should be no trouble for any intern whose work has been satisfactory to obtain a residency. They are going to need 250 interns and 200 residents. There are to be 2,900 beds and 8,000 outpatients to be cared for daily. There are to be 54 operating rooms, which will be supplied with sterile air. There is to be a loudspeaker system by which the operator can talk directly to the pathologist, to whom specimens are sent by means of a pneumatic tube system.

Some "dream come true," isn't it? Also, they are to give the residents master's degrees at the end of the service. Who says the South is backward? They are slow, all right, but La. has really stepped up lately.

Until Monday—when we can really speak to each other. Be sure and talk lots, so I can enjoy hearing your voice.

Love,
Alice

Oмана

Monday, February 14

My Dearest Alice:

Can it be possible that I talked to you tonight? It seemed that you were so near and that I could just reach out and touch you. Or perhaps that you were at the apartment at 603 SW 1st St. in Rochester and I was at 849 SW 1st. And I had so much to tell you and I seemed to be at a loss of words—"A dream come true." A few minutes of pleasure to last for many months. Now I cannot study tonight.

What a weekend for outcalls. My partner left town so I had all of the calls in northwest Omaha, and some of the streets are very difficult to find. And practically all of the patients are Works Progress Administration employees and their families.

I am going "bats" on climatology. Printed about 100 maps that I plan to use in the thesis. Yes, everything is due to climate. Even the fact that I get good reception from distant Salt Lake City on my radio tonight must be due to some climatic factor, since I rarely get it this early.

You tell that unruly patient of yours that he is very lucky to have you as his physician. Could I change places with him? But I know that an incident like that will not discourage you. All the more courage to conquer unforeseen difficulties.

Isn't it a thrill to accomplish some work that no one else has done before (remember Dr. MacCarty?). I had planned a major part of my thesis for some of my own research, but now I find that someone has already done the work. A change in the outline, a new chapter, and now for some original work.

We have some of the alumni and their wives over for dinner Friday again. Handshakes, bridge—and then they all assure us that they had a good time. Well, I always do, and I feel that it promotes a better relationship between alumnus and active. I hope to get a Nu Sigma Nu Alumni Wives Club organized. Wish us luck.

You probably wonder if we ever study. Frankly, we have very little class work—most of the periods are clinics. But they still give examinations at the end of the year.

Charity must be a grand place. Too bad I could not intern there.

I still think that I am dreaming when I recall that I talked to you tonight. Dream or reality, it was a great pleasure.

Love,
Joe

NEW ORLEANS
Mon nite, Feb. 14
8 o'clock

Dearest Joe—

I had been looking forward to tonight since Thursday and when it came—oh, I just can't express my feelings. Your voice sounded so nice—it's such a nice crisp voice. I haven't heard anything like it for so long—and gee, it made me want to see you oh so very much. What a grand thing the telephone is—and the television which they say is coming will really be wonderful. But it surely can't take the place of the actual presence. Now, when I look at your picture I can hear your voice again, and then I get so happy I want to dance a jig! This has certainly been the most perfect valentine anyone could have.

Dot just came by to see me. She said she thought I'd want someone to talk to after the phone call she had heard so much about. I talked about you so much that she's very anxious to meet this perfect medical student. I assured her I wasn't exaggerating a mite when I spoke of all your good points. In fact, I couldn't say half enough.

I catch myself just stopping everything and sitting up, my pen in my hand—just staring into space—but dreaming such nice things. I really think it is a downright shame when people want to be near enough to at least see each other occasionally. But every time I start thinking that, I remind myself how fortunate I am to have met you at all—and especially have your friendship. Gee, I surely can't complain.

You should hear how the other patients on the ward, the nurses, and the interns talk of my patient, the race track groom. When I found out that he has lice tonight, I decided that must be the chief thing the matter with him. I surely wish he would leave the hospital, but he told me tonight he was going to stay another month.

Your cases surely sound interesting. It must be quite educational to make visits to the home as you do. Do you go alone or does another student or an instructor accompany you?

I'm so interested in Dr. Stastny. I'm surely going to the breakfast for Dr. Mabel Akin, the president of the National Women's Medical Association, now. Most probably Dr. Akin will know her. I hope I can meet her some day.

Have you ever read the true story of Longfellow's Evangeline? You know, she found her Gabriel just a few miles from here on the banks of the Bayou Teche under a large old live oak tree. The tree and the chapel where they worshipped are still standing—and really well worth your visiting. Near them also is the old home of Joe Jefferson, the inspiration for the brand name of our Jefferson Island Salt. There are several salt mines near here which were certainly interesting to me. I wonder if I'm putting my idea across. The radio says "Let's waltz for old time's sake" and I second the motion.

As the telephone conversation seemed so very short, so is the limit of letter writing finally reached. I close with the anticipation of hearing a certain "Yankee" voice in my dreams tonight.

Thanks again for making me the happiest gal on St. Valentine's Day—

Love,
Alice

OMAHA

Thursday, Feb. 17

My Dearest Alice:

Again I was so very anxious to receive your letter and thoroughly enjoyed it. Yes, telephone or television cannot take the place of actual presence. All the fellows have heard so much about you that they do not believe that such a girl medical student can exist. Of course you will meet Dr. Stastny whenever you come to Omaha. She also attends most of the conventions of the National Women's Medical Association.

Talk about dreaming—I had a very pleasant one the other night. I went to the Mardi Gras primarily to see you. And I can still recall the details of your room. And the good time that we had. But what a disappointment to feel a sudden jerking and have A.C. say, "Joe, it's twenty to eight." Yes, I was still in the trance when I got to class.

We are having an epidemic of colds on outcall. I have five down at the children's home—it is like making daily ward rounds at the hospital. Now all that we need is an isolation ward there, but they are so crowded that I am afraid we have to continue using one corner of the room for isolation.

Theoretically, two students go on outcalls together, but recently we have been so busy that we go alone. On many occasions our ingenuity is taxed to the utmost when we have to make use of some of the meager facilities available in some of the homes. And on many occasions, I wished that I had listened a little more attentively to lectures on infectious diseases or Therapeutics. And then to make the decision whether the case should be hospitalized or not, or whether to call in a staff man—more fun. At least it makes us rely upon our own judgement and gives us some confidence in ourselves. Nevertheless, I have been careful to do all the necessary examinations and tests and never to overdose.

One case that I saw today certainly irritated me. The mother is just recovering from pneumonia and still has some pleuritis, but she had to get up and clean house. Her three grown daughters were too busy reading and listening to the radio to do it.

110 maps completed for my thesis—I am convinced that climate is a great factor in disease (even headache, toothache, etc.). Now if I can only convince the readers of that. I must experience the climate of New Orleans someday—I have written so much about it—barometric variability, maximum & minimum temperature, climatic stimulation, rainfall, etc.

I must see the places that you described in your letter—but could we have one evening just to sit and talk?

Another long wait until Monday.

Love,

Joe

NEW ORLEANS

Thu Nite, Feb. 17

Dearest Joe—

My favorite patient, the groom, was discharged today, much to the relief of the other patients on the ward and myself. He made the intern so angry that he discharged him before he had intended to, but the results of his G.I. series were negative. Which seems to prove what the intern had believed all the time—that there was really nothing wrong with him at all.

Your fraternity certainly must have a good spirit of companionship. I think that some social contact between physicians and students means so much, for there is so much to the art and practice of medicine that cannot be learned from textbooks, and only an experienced physician can smooth the way for a young M.D. just starting out.

I hear—by rumor—that our State Board exams are to be over by June 5th. I'm surely hoping I'll be all through by the time you come down. In fact, I'm already bewailing the fact that internship necessarily will make your visit much too short.

We have had no definite word from AEI as to where we are to be initiated, but they say they hope it will be before March so we can send a delegate to the National Convention in April. Best of luck in your work on the thesis.

Love,
Alice

NEW ORLEANS
Mon Nite, Feb. 21

Dearest Joe—

You certainly are fortunate in the way you have to manage your outcalls. I can't imagine the hospital here really letting us decide anything definitely for ourselves. And I surely feel that loss, too, for I fear I might be sadly lacking at an emergency. That is one reason I so prefer to intern here. There must be so much more for us to learn from our instructors during our intern year. All of us students have been complaining because we have been given so little therapeutic. Our professors reply, "You'll get that during your internship." And now another rumor is afloat that if 2 or 3 of our present interns don't get busy, they won't be given their diploma at the end of the year. They really mean it when they call our internship our fifth year of Medicine. Do you get your M.D. degree this June, or just a Bachelor of Medicine as we do?

I surprised the folks this weekend. They've been pretty lonesome lately, especially since Uncle left. I surely enjoy walking in on them when they're not expecting me! Have you been home recently? I haven't heard about Dennis for quite a while.

It is just starting to rain, so I suppose we'll have a return of spring. We've had quite a cold snap. There was frost on the ground for the last two mornings.

We plan to have our sorority meeting early Friday so we may attend the Parade of Hermes later.

Love,
Alice

OMAHA
Tuesday morning, Feb. 22

My Dearest Alice:

I hope that you excuse this late letter, but the books from Mayo's were due last night and I stayed up until I finished them. Needless to say, I obtained very little sleep.

And now G.I. dispensary. Dr. J.D. McCarthy has not arrived yet, and I am hoping that he will not come for an hour or so. This gastro-enterology is an elective dispensary service and I am taking it during outcall.

We just had another snow last night—about 3 inches of soft, fluffy flakes. And now the sun will come out, to make candid photography in the snow a pleasure.

Colds, colds, colds and more colds. Eleven children in bed at the home last Friday. As long as scarlet fever does not start, everything will be OK.

Had some Bohemian patients on outcall yesterday. They thought it was swell that I could talk their language—although I must say that I need a little brushing up on my grammar.

Do you ever listen to any Neb. radio stations? All we hear now is

"Nebraska—the white spot of the Nation—no sales or luxury tax, bonded indebtedness, etc." They are making a campaign to attract new industries to the state.

I have been trying to get a N.O. station on my radio but so far have been able to get only one. Perhaps we need a new radio.

Sorry—here comes McCarthy.

10 a.m. (in library)

What an hour of lectures. "Never mind the patients, just listen to me" is Dr. McCarthy's attitude, but he does give some very good lectures. "Keep your ears pinned back or someone will knock them back," etc.—all included in a lecture on Osteoarthritis of the spine being confused with gastric ulcer and inflammation of the gallbladder.

And now we came to the hospital to see an atypical case of pernicious anemia, and when I mentioned that it might be a carcinoma of the gastro-intestinal tract—well, you can guess what happened. Dr. McCarthy said that C.A. never resembles P.A. picture. But I maintained that I saw some blood pictures this summer that did. MacCarty vs. McCarthy.

For original work on my thesis, I plan to correlate our recent polio epidemic with meteorological conditions and—now, don't laugh—but I do believe that the oscillations of a manic depressive may be due to climatic stimulation and a dozen other things. Now to prove or disprove it. Perhaps I will turn into a meteorologist.

Back to reality—I am late to class.

Love,
Joe

NEW ORLEANS

Thurs. Nite, Feb. 24

Dearest Joe—

I just got back from the first Mardi Gras parade. It was the parade
of Momus and the theme was "Legends." I enjoyed Ali Baba and
"Perseus and the Sea Serpent" especially. The floats were very pretty
tonight. They are drawn by horses. We got quite chilly.

Your Dr. McCarthy sounds as if he is a typical Medical professor.
Our expression down here is "Don't stick out your neck if you don't
want it chopped off." It's too bad he hasn't had a course under Dr.
MacCarty. I just seethe inside whenever they mention him down here
and then say they don't agree with him. Having seen his work, his
specimens, and having listened to his lectures, I believe he's all there.

Meteorological conditions are something I know absolutely nothing about. You're way above my head, but if you say there's something to it, I don't doubt you. As Dr. MacCarty would say, I have no
right to an opinion, knowing nothing about the subject, but at least
I know that if it holds your attention, I'm all for it.

Louis Armstrong is now "tooting" away. No, I've never had a
Nebraska station. My radio must not be such a good one either. But
I'm going to keep on trying.

Nebraska sounds like the taxpayer's paradise. I hear we're to have
a general 2¢ sales tax as soon as it passes the legislature. It has been
called a luxury tax and was double within N.O. limits. However,
there have been many objections.

I hate to close a letter to you, for it seems almost like being with
you when I write you and read your letters. Goodnight, my dear.

Love,

Alice

NEW ORLEANS
Mon. Nite, Feb. 28

Dearest Joe—

I waited until I got back from the Mardi Gras ball tonight to write
to you for I thought you might be interested in it. The balls are held
at the Municipal Auditorium, and the crowd starts coming at seven
o'clock to be sure and get a seat—and tonight, it didn't even begin
until about ten o'clock. The parade ends at the Auditorium, and all the
maskers from the float then enter the building for a good time. The
queen and her maids entered first. They were beautifully gowned—all
in white—and each carried a huge bouquet of red American beau-
ties. The queen was quite pretty, and her long green velvet and ermine
train was really a beautiful sight. Then the curtain rose on King Pro-
teus and all his court. He was dressed in gold with a long sparkling
train, and after several promenades, so everyone could see his splen-
dor, the queen joined him on a throne of the prettiest shade of blue.
All was quite formal and sedate until all these ceremonies were over.
Then the members of the king's court—very fancifully dressed in
everything from silk overalls to highland Scottish kilts—were turned
loose, and when they started, the fun began.

The orchestra leader, who had very primly been playing the
"Spring Song," swung into "The Big Apple" and the call-outs began.
Each member of the court selected his call-out and after another
short promenade, with presentations to the king and queen, they
had their dance. It was quite a unique picture—lovely gowned ladies
dancing with farmers, clowns, knights, old ladies, etc. However, we
left soon after this for I, for one, soon get enough of having to sit
still and watch other people dance.

I haven't seen any parades since the one I wrote you about Thursday night. I wanted to see the children's parade Sat. noon, but didn't
get out of school in time. However, I hope to see most of them tomorrow. King Zulu, the Negro king, is the most amusing, and then Rex

himself parades at about noon. All the city has been asked to mask for the big day tomorrow, and fun and merriment will hold sway.

It seems that I miss you more each day, if possible, and no doubt, you would be surprised at some of the places where I think of you— by the bedside during ward rounds, when Dr. Wilder's work on hyperinsulinism is quoted, when I see some beautiful sight, as the azaleas abloom along our flower trail—

My love,
Alice

OMAHA
Monday, Feb. 28
5:30

My Dearest Alice:

I just returned from basketball practice and if my penmanship is more unsteady than usual, blame it on general muscular fatigue. There is nothing like being in good physical condition, and I need a few more practices to remove some extra adipose tissue—yes, all of 158 lbs.

The mailman is certainly my pal today—twice—once for bringing the Times-Picayune and again for bringing your letter, although I enjoyed the latter the best. I have read all about the Mardi Gras in the Times. It must be unforgettable and someday I will see it. Would it not be fun—parades, balls, and all the time you at my side. Anything connected with New Orleans is tops with me.

Incidentally, I went home this weekend. It seemed like months since I visited there. Mother had a cold and I made her stay indoors. I hope it does not get any worse but with forcing fluids, rest, etc., she should recover soon. I am still looking for a cure for sinusitis that she has not tried—perhaps change of climate.

Dennis is cuter than ever. In fact he sits up himself already.

Surprise—I brought Nellie back with me. It is just like old times in Rochester, but we need you to make it complete. A ride to Silver Lake, to Mayo Park, out to the Institute and then to the Valencia.

There is the dinner bell.

10:00 p.m.

Just returned from outcall—saw six cases and what an experience. One of my chronic gall bladder cases is a constant source of trouble. First she would not diet (she weighs over 200) and now she complains of fainting spells coming on in bed 10–20 times a day and, to accommodate me, she had one on suggestion. Pulse regular—respiration & blood pressure normal—no loss of pupillary reflexes and other signs indicative of hysteria. A little psychotherapy and perhaps some luminal will stop the attacks (so I told her). Now for an experiment—tomorrow I will give her a tablet of calcium bicarbonate and convince her that she will have no more attacks.

One more month of outcall. We do learn a lot of bedside manners and in some cases how to get along without drugs when the family cannot purchase them and we are not allowed to dispense them. More problems.

I had an interesting experience last Friday. I was called out of Neuropsychiatry class to interview a patient. It seemed that an old man strayed into the admitting room and did not know where or who he was. With a little German & more Bohemian I got his history and had a psychiatry clinic of my own—a senile dementia.

Now to read more about Mardi Gras. Until Thursday—my love,

Joe

New Orleans

Fri. Nite, March 4

Dearest Joe—

This has been quite a week. I managed to squeeze on Canal Street to see the Parade. It was some sight. Many of the people were masked, many very fantastically, and every one was in a good humor and making friends with everyone else. I tried to get some pictures, but most of them turned out to be fade-outs. There was such a mob that I couldn't do much with my box camera, but I enjoyed the fun of taking them anyway.

I missed the night parade and Rex ball. That surgery quiz came at a very inconvenient time. Wednesday we were on emergency service until 10—and of course I got a case at 5 o'clock. They say Tuesday (Mardi Gras day) was such a busy one that they couldn't even keep a record of all those they treated. Wed. nite we saw two interesting operations. One mental patient had jumped from a window of Hotel Dieu Hospital in an attempt at suicide. When it didn't work, he stabbed himself in the abdomen seven times that afternoon. He only perforated the intestine in one place, however, and is still living. Then we saw a colored girl who was shot in the abdomen.

These pictures I'm enclosing are the best of my bunch. I'm hoping to get some of King Zulu for you.

Mother is going to make my intern suits for me, and she sent me the first one today, for criticism. I'm quite thrilled over it—and hope I'm not being presumptuous in having them made. Won't it be a thrill to be the "Men in White."

I'm so glad it won't be long until Monday.

My love,

Alice

OMAHA
Thursday, March 10
9:15 a.m.

My Darling:

Today I must spend all of the time organizing my thesis. Imagine, I have ceased reading articles and writing it already. So far I have traced Climatology from pre-historic times through China, India, Mesopotamia, Egypt, Greece, and Rome and have just started on the Christian era. Do you think that I can cover the remaining 1,900 years in the next month?

Nellie is behaving nicely, but she would love to have you as a driver. Would not that be grand!

Our spring is gone and I fear that winter will start again. More trouble for my sinuses. Do you know of any "sure-cure" remedy—or are there any in medicine? I plan to enlist in the ROTC medical corps, the main reason being that an officer can ride horseback any afternoon at Council Bluffs and receive service credit for it. And the first chance we get, you and I will go on that moonlight ride.

My father and mother plan to come to Omaha Monday. Mother is much better now. Dennis had a cold—but what child does not?—much to the worry of his mother.

I bet that you will be glad when surgical service will be over—about like me with outcall, although I have learned a lot on it. Received another call this morning—perhaps another cold, rheumatic heart, or what-not.

Sometimes I wonder just how you find it possible to read my letters—but they all mean I miss you very, very, much.

With love,
Joe

New Orleans

Thurs Nite, March 10

Dearest Joe—

I'm getting more and more anxious to read your thesis. However, I'm afraid I'm going to need help in understanding it. May I have some personal instructions, please sir?

We have really had a spring day. Even the medico-eds blossomed out in spring dresses. It's grand weather now but I'm already hoping it won't get too warm too soon. It gets almost unbearably warm here in New Orleans during the summer. This will be the first summer I won't be able to spend it at home, in the country. I think I'll invest my first month's check of perhaps $8—I hope—on an electric fan.

Do you think Sept. is the proper time to apply for fellowships? I thought maybe we should apply earlier—as in June. Do you know if they have a special fellowship in Gynecology and Obstetrics or is that incorporated in the surgery fellowship? I think I should like some special training in those lines.

I phoned my folks last night as I hadn't heard from them for a few days. Mother had big news and said she was planning to call me later. It seems my folks are going to move. We had been living, as you know, at the Veterans Hospital, which is four miles from Alex. The building we are living in is sadly in need of repair, but the gov't refused to fix it as they have been going to demolish it with several others for the last 4 or 5 years. And it has always been much too small for us, especially for a family who loves company as mine do. So we're moving into town. I'm delighted and am just hoping the folks will be satisfied. I'm sure Mother will like it much better but it might take Dad farther from his favorite fishing hole.

Sinus trouble is really a problem, isn't it? I hope your Mother is faring better now.

My love,
Alice

OMAHA
Monday, March 14
6:45

My Darling Alice:

I am on anesthetics this week. Three of us get to assist in administering the anesthesia for the surgery. I hope to learn something on this service because so far the only anesthetic that I gave was ether by the drip method & open mask on a home OB, accompanied with some oral anesthesia. Intravenous is not used here as much as at Mayo's.

Business is on the up & up—measles & one bronchopneumonia yesterday. I wonder what my calls will be tonight. And now it is time to go. Until later—

9:00 p.m.

Three cases of measles—with typical Koplik's spots and everything. A patient 80 years old with vomiting & diarrhea, high blood pressure, and very emaciated. My bet is on a G.I. carcinoma.

I saw the pictures of the Mardi Gras in Life. It certainly must have been a glorious spectacle. Mother took home some of the Times-Picayune you sent to read more about it.

We had a rare treat in class last Friday. One of the fellows, a habitual somnambulist, fell asleep, got up, walked to the front of the amphitheater, in front of the professor, up the steps and awoke when he came to the door. I know, that sounds awfully rare, but it certainly was funny to see him return to his seat very, very embarrassed.

Rats—another outcall—6 years old, vomiting, diarrhea, convulsions, and about 4–5 miles out. Wish me luck.

10:15 p.m.

What a call—Nellie and I roared down Creighton Blvd. breaking every traffic law, hitting bumps, etc., and then we found no 3635 Taylor St. Instead it was in East Omaha—out of my territory. At times like this we would like to call the University operator and give him hell, but perhaps it is better to follow Dale Carnegie, politely informing him of the mistake, and as it happened, it was the fault of the patient's mother. Blame it all on the excitement not the climate this time.

About the Mayo fellowships. I think it would be nice to have them start Oct. 1, 1939, and apply a year ahead of time. Or is it easier to get in on July 1st—we must find out about that. I believe that they do have a fellowship in OB and Gyn, but I will find out for certain. Have you definitely decided to take this specialty? So far I have planned to take internal medicine. Alice, no matter how, we must get to Rochester next year.

In view of developments abroad, I wonder how long Czechoslovakia will maintain its independence. However, they will not give up without a struggle. They are usually slow to make up their minds, but once convinced, they never stop in spite of all odds. Let us hope that Hitler stays away from there.

I hope to see your new home this summer. And the fishing hole. Reminds me of the times that I went fishing near Clarkson—and what a thrill when I caught a bull-head.

Nellie & I are more lonely for you everyday. Imagine, 6 fellows in our room tonight—including one alumnus & two town actives— and clothes are all over the place. All that I ask is a place to write a letter to you. All the beds in the dorm are taken.

With love,

Joe

NEW ORLEANS
Thurs Nite, March 17

Dearest Joe—

A very long week has come to a very happy climax. This has certainly been my lucky day. I found out this noon that I was among the lucky third of the surgical section who are to be exempt from the final surgical practical. Then I came home to find a new dress Mother had sent me—plus, best of all, a letter from you, to make the day a perfect one.

Did I ever tell you how I enjoy your letters? I'm sure I haven't halfway told you how I do. Believe me, this year has been the happiest of my life because of your friendship.

I was supposed to be on for anesthesia this week but was also scheduled for metabolic clinic during the same hours, so the anesthesia had to be postponed. Ether by the drip method is the only anesthesia we have the opportunity to give.

The radio says "I miss you more than ever before," taking the words right from the tip of my tongue or pen!

Ah—I agree with you that we must get to Rochester next year. Every time I think of it I am thrilled—and half scared that something will happen so that I won't get to make it. Oh, how I hope for it. It is the acme of my ambitions, and I don't even think about after that. Here's hoping our dreams will come true.

To tell you the truth, I can't seem to decide just what kind of graduate work I prefer. Each branch of medicine (excepting dermatology) is so very interesting—and internal medicine is without doubt the best fundamental branch. But there is nothing which infuriates me so as a poorly managed delivery. It brings, I believe, the most heartbreak—and joy—this obstetrics practice does. And, ahem, pathology is supposed to be a good field for women. I wish I were a more determined sort and could make up my mind definitely as to which and what I should plan on.

Isn't Hitler trying to become "master of all he surveys"—and more! His accession of Austria has certainly been a brutal step. I certainly do hope he stays away from Czechoslovakia. He's done enough harm in Germany.

I wish your mother and you could see our flower show which is opening next week. It's always so lovely. I'm going to try to persuade Mother to return with me Sunday. She would enjoy the flower show and opera "La Traviata," which the LSU musical school is to present here Tues nite. Wish we could all enjoy it together.

With love,
Alice

NEW ORLEANS
Mon. Nite, March 21

Dearest Joe—

I've been looking forward to your letter so much. All the while I was home this weekend I kept wishing I could hear from you. Oh, I'm so anxious for you to come down here and especially to meet my folks. I talk about you so much they feel almost as if they know you. We had a very grand weekend, even though it did try to rain me out. It seems that Alexandria has a very low altitude—and very poor drainage. The street in front of our new home (we hope) was a veritable lake. How I would like to be home when the time comes to move. I'd love the job of "fixing" everything as I thought it should go. So I had to control myself with picking out which room, furniture, etc., should be mine.

We have to wait for permission from Washington, D.C., to move. Ahem! Aren't we important! Gee, there is more red tape to old Uncle Sam's business!

Wouldn't it be grand if we could just push a button and reverse to any part of our lives we would like to live over? If we could, I know I would spend most of my time with Nellie and her driver seeing Rochester—Ooh—they're playing "Memories" and that always gets me, especially since this summer.

Honestly, I can't understand how you stand reading all this raving of mine. I have always wished for someone who would be a real pal—whom I could talk with about anything and everything and share my most treasured moments with, thus making them all the more precious. And so it seems, you've had the role forced on you. And you have added more to it than I could ever have dreamed of. And, as one is never satisfied, now I wish I could at least see and talk with you at times. Ah, what a month June will be!

While home I found these pictures. The view of the hospital in Pineville is similar to that to be seen from our present front porch. Dad works in the building to the extreme right in the picture. It is the colored building and practically a complete hospital in itself.

Pineville is a small town just across Red River from Alexandria. Isn't that a dreary looking picture? The levee broke above Alex, and lots of the lowlands between the break and Alex are flooded like this. I suppose the majority of the land is uncultivated and not densely populated. I'm so glad the hospital is on a hill!

It's thundering outside. Our April showers are a bit early. Now I start looking toward Thursday.

> Love,
> Alice

OMAHA

Wednesday night, March 23

My Darling:

What an eventful day, starting off with a letter from you. Imagine, I received it 18 hours after it was postmarked.

My father and mother came to town again this forenoon—and now comes the big surprise, something that I shall never forget. My parents took me to the DeBrown Auto Sales Co. and asked, "Which do you prefer, black, sky blue, Biltmore tan or green?" What a surprise. A car for my graduation—and, above all, a 1938 Studebaker Commander. The decision—a coupe in Biltmore tan. What a dream, with a radio and everything. I cannot understand how I deserve such a gift. I can hardly wait until next week when the car will be delivered from the factory. I am ever so sorry that you cannot be here to have the first ride in it with me. And christen it. Do you have any names that you can suggest? Please help me find one.

But, gee, it will be difficult to part with Nancy. We have been together for almost two years now, and in spite of a few escapades where she broke for me when we were miles from nowhere, she has always done her best. In snow, mud, ice, emergency trips to see a patient or just for pleasure trips, Nancy was always ready. And many winter mornings she was the only Nu Sig car that started. But things do grow old and must make room for posterity.

Received a communication from my friend Dr. I. Rutledge of the Clinic. He published "Criteria for the Diagnosis of Presumptive Gout," Proceedings of the Staff Meetings of the Mayo Clinic, Vol. 12 P 189 Mar 1937, and I have not had the opportunity to look it up yet. I bet Ivan is one of Dr. Hench's disciples. Incidentally, Dr. Hench is in England now reporting his results on treatment of arthritis with jaundice.

About having the role of your pal forced on me—I desire it, I welcome it with open arms. I, too, have wanted a real friend, someone with whom I can converse, philosophize, dance, and share my happiest moments. Now, it is only by letter, but what happiness they bring. It was only six weeks this summer, but I feel that I have known you for years and years.

Gee, what a day—and am I enthused about my new car. You must see it.

Mother sends her regards.

And now, sweet dreams of you.

Love,

Joe

New Orleans

Mon. Nite, March 28

My dearest—

I'm so happy for you. Isn't it grand? A new car, and a Studebaker at that! The young Dr. Holoubek is really starting in style. Gee, I know it must have given your parents a lot of joy to give you a nice gift like that. Well might they be proud of their son! And oh, how I'd like to listen to that radio by our lake in Rochester. I do hope that you think of me just once when you drive it the first time—selfish me!

Today was our first on OB duty. We were very fortunate, Dot and I, having a delivery each. Hers was the first case. Unfortunately, it was a precipitate delivery, and she only got to tie the cord and deliver the placenta, but she says she is much more confident now. My patient had a prolapsed bladder, and we feared she would get a cervical tear. Fortunately, everything went well. I tried the Ritgen method and didn't push as hard as I pulled (or pushed upward), and the head popped out too soon. "That's the way you get lacerations." "Yes, sir." And was I glad she hadn't torn.

It was a little girl, and, surprise, the mother asked me my name. So I have an honest-to-goodness namesake. Jeanne Alice DuPont! Naturally, she's the prettiest baby on the newborn ward! Ahem!

Please send my regards to your folks. It was so nice of your mother to remember me. I'm so anxious to meet them both. And do remember to remind yourself that someone is missing you terribly.

Alice

When may I have a picture of the new car? I'm making a study of the name most suitable!

OMAHA
Mon. night, March 28

Darling:

Another night spent on my thesis. For the last two weeks I have been writing every night, and tonight I am proofreading the first two chapters. Gosh, I wish this would be over. It seems weeks & months since I could think of anything else but climate, meteorology, and spas. After April 8th at least I will be able to get some sleep.

My car came Saturday but it will not be ready until tomorrow. What a dream. But, gee, I wish that you would be here to ride in it with me.

Before I forget, our spring vacation is from April 1–6, so please send my next Monday's letter to Clarkson. I may have to return the 5th in order to paste some maps into my thesis. However, I plan to go home for Easter, too.

Imagine, 70 more days until graduation. When and where do you graduate? We have our exercises at Lincoln. It would be time for a celebration, but I will wait until I get to N.O.—or will it be Alexandria?

Our spring weather has changed into fog, and I hope that it does not develop into sleet by the morning. But we do need rain.

It's past midnight and tonight I must go to bed. Friday I decided to stay up all night to write—but never again.

With treasured memories of the past and great hopes for the future—

>All my love,
>Joe

NEW ORLEANS
Thu. Afternoon, March 31
On OB Ward

Dearest Joe—

Isn't air mail a great improvement? I was so glad to get your letter last night. I was anxious to hear more about the new car. I suppose that by now, you are great friends. I've been thinking about a name for it. Have you decided on one yet? Since you seem to go in for names starting with "N" for your automobiles, how about Nola? I'm hoping that will prove an appropriate name, as I am hoping to get acquainted with it in N.O., La.

This OB service is all right when we can do deliveries, but we seem to spend most of our time doing urinalyses. However, we've had two deliveries each, which isn't so bad. We're expecting to see an abnormal tonight. The woman is 29 years old, a primipara, with a slightly narrowed outlet. She's been in labor over 48 hours and is as yet only 2 fingers dilated. Our class decided that a Caesarian section should be done, but our chief, Dr. Phillips John Carter, is always conservative and is still waiting. The presentation is right occiput posterior, and her membranes ruptured prematurely. They are debating, I believe, as to whether a section should be done if nothing else develops. I surely hope they do something soon for she's really been suffering, even though they've been giving her hypnotics.

I suppose that by now the thesis is practically completed. You really undertook a huge job, and I know it has been most excellently done. I am really anxious to know your conclusions.

As to that long anticipated time of graduation—our exercises are held in Baton Rouge, usually about June 2. What a celebration we'll have. Gee, it's a pleasure to look forward to it. I suppose we'll have to extend the celebration over Alexandria and New Orleans, too, won't we? You must visit both places.

I'm sure you'll have a nice vacation. Do make the most of it—and I'm looking for some pictures. Give my best regards to your folks, your sister, and that big boy Dennis—and to yourself.

> Love,
> Alice

CLARKSON
Sunday, April 3

My Darling:

We had a family reunion today—I have not eaten so much for months and months—kolaches and all of the other tasty foods that Mother makes. And you should see Dennis—my, it has been three months since I saw him last, and he is practically a man already— all of 23 lbs.—much too active and fortunately he does not cry. Apparently he does not take after his uncle. He has had only a slight cold this winter and otherwise is OK. You should see him smile—he makes everyone happy.

Nola is the name. How very appropriate. So far she has 299.5 miles on—and not a scratch. I hope that none develops for several months. Everyone wants a ride in it.

Imagine, I have spent two whole days without having to think of my thesis—much. It will bother me from Tue. to Fri. and then it will be handed in—whoopee.

You may find that I exaggerated quite freely on my climatological theories—but Uncle Mac says that that is the only way to teach. And, furthermore, I want to arouse interest in the subject, & what better way is there to do it than by stimulating an argument.

Right now if I could be in the same room with you, see your face, hear your voice & touch your hand—there would be no happier man in the world.

With all my love,
Joe

OMAHA
Friday, April 8

My Dearest:

At last my thesis is completed and handed in—an hour before the required time. 275 pages—125 figures. I cannot believe it, actually completed. Incidentally, the title is "Observations in Meteorology & Meteoropathology." We have to present the original copy to the college library, but I have a carbon copy that you may read if you choose to sometime.

Another surprise—we just had a snowball fight. Yes, we have some snow again. Tuesday night it rained, followed by sleet & 4 inches of snow. What a change after the warm weather we had had. However, this will be gone in a few days & spring may be here to stay.

And tomorrow is the day of your AEI initiation. Another one of your ambitions realized. Congratulations. I am certain that you will realize your next ambition—to get a fellowship at Mayo's. Right?

You get a vacation for Easter while we do not. However, I plan to skip my Saturday morning classes and go home Friday night.

Spring "rushing" season is on now, & we must go to Lincoln to contact the pre-meds who are coming over next year. Too bad we are not on the same campus.

I still cannot believe it. My thesis is finished. No more working all night, and more time to write to you.

Love,
Joe

New Orleans
Saturday, April 9

Dearest Joe—

I am so thrilled I just can't wait to write to you. We've just been initiated into Alpha Epsilon Iota. It was a very impressive ceremony, and everyone is very enthused. We selected a fine group of girls for officers of our new sorority and are hoping we are off to a good start. Isn't it a fine thing to belong to a grand national fraternal organization—to feel that you have many friends over the entire United States and can be proud of every one of them? The boys have been very nice, sending us congratulation telegrams. Now, at last, we shall be represented in the Interfraternity Council.

Mon. Nite

Well, as you see, I was interrupted. Dot spent Sat. nite with me and was fussing for me to hurry to bed. At least I got my raving about the fraternity off my mind.

Nola is such a pretty young thing, I'm wondering if I should be jealous! Really, she is a beauty and I know you're very proud of her. At least you certainly should be. Ah, but Dennis is surely a fine looking little man. He looks as if he's about to pop out with some bright saying.

Gretchen is on OB duty this week, so with Dot away and Alice Tisdale in California at the AEI convention, I'm trying to hold up the feminine side of the class. It's quite a job to withstand all the teasing and jibes without someone to share it with, but I believe I can take it by now!

I have a very sweet little patient, 13 years old, in Gynecology. She's been having heavy bleeding for almost a year. She is from the central part of the state, and came to the hospital alone. She had been crying when I went to see her this afternoon and said she was lonesome. Gee, I felt sorry for her. I asked her what she wanted to read and she said anything but preferably fairy tales—and nothing with love in it! I laughed—and am now trying to locate some fairy tales.

I was just looking at your pictures of Nola again. That surely is a swell-looking car—and very becoming to you.

Mother mentioned again in her letter today how she wanted to meet you and your folks. Ah, what a month—June—and until then, dreams and anticipation.

Love,
Alice

Omaha
Tuesday morning, April 12
Before class

Darling:

My thesis was checked over by the committee and returned yesterday for me to have it bound. This gave me a splendid opportunity to revise a few pages and change it a little. And now finally it is being bound into book form and I am through—I hope. Now for about 24 hours more of good sleep. It seems that the more that I sleep, the sleepier I get. Perhaps I was accustomed to only 5–6 hrs.

I was out at the Home last night and have a ward full of acute tonsils. For weeks we have been trying to have them taken out, and it will finally be done next week. Next I have to do routine physicals again. I will hate to leave the kids this summer, but I plan to get the appointment for A.C. so that I could keep in touch with them—at least indirectly.

Only about 55 more days. State Boards two months from tomorrow. It has been rumored that one of the Board members stated that we should not study for them. All that I need is a confirmation of that statement & my books will close. But a review of my medical work would help my short memory.

Now to work—and for you—my love,

Joe

ALEXANDRIA
Fri. Nite, April 15

Dearest Joe—

It surely is a pleasure to be at home, with nothing to do except eat, sleep, fix my room, pay a few calls, and—best of all—have Easter dinner with some very dear friends of ours. The Tysons have a baby, John Charles, about 8 months old, and he's quite the master of all he surveys. He's trying to start walking, but anxious parents are afraid it is too soon and are holding him back, much to his disgust. Babies born last August must be extraordinarily brilliant, don't you agree?

Yes, we've been having grand spring weather, too, but it began to look cloudy this afternoon, and tonight the wind is very strong and the radio terrible—a pretty good sign of trouble ahead. I surely hope all is serene again for Easter morning.

I think our new home is very satisfactory, and I like every bit of it. After 10 years on a government reservation, it's as if we were visiting to finally be in a real house. We have so much more room that we almost get lost from one another. And Mother left my room for me to fix, so I'm getting the fun of moving myself. Gee, but do I have a lot of pure junk. I made quite an effort and threw away a lot of it, but I'm afraid I still have a lot of unnecessary items—but I can't bear to throw them away.

Your state boards are very late, aren't they? I think we get through ours on the 4th of June. How I wish you did, too.

It is nice for you to spend Easter at home. I know you and your family had a happy time and I hope all the joys and blessings of Easter remain with you always—

Love, Alice

Western Union

MISS ALICE BAKER
1733 WHITE ST

LOVING EASTER GREETINGS AND TENDEREST
MEMORIES OF YOU.

JOE HOLOUBEK

OMAHA
Wednesday, April 27
10 p.m.

Darling:

More April showers—we had four of them today—but Nola is safe in the garage.

I cannot believe it. I have been studying—and hard. Imagine. Completed my Bio-chem and now Pharmacology, the only course that I disliked. Perhaps because of the instructor.

Dr. Perrin Long of Johns Hopkins gave us a lecture on sulfanilamide this morning. From his observations, we are wasting it by trying it on lobar pneumonia. However, Nebraska is not as bad as one of the eastern hospitals where a patient is given prontylin on admittance & if he does not recover within 5 days, they do a history & physical. You don't have to believe that—it is one of those rumors.

"LIGHTS OUT EVERYBODY"—My room is full. The lights will go out, and just for another crazy radio program. I'd rather hear Wayne King & write to you.

Later

What a program. And now A.C. wants to go out, so to Jameison's Buffet for some beer.

11:30

And they say that beer is a stimulant. But tonight it is very thrilling—perhaps the weather, 40° above, might have something to do with it.

Incidentally, I was quite surprised when I read the Sunday Omaha World Herald and found some quotations from my thesis. It seems that one reporter had spring fever and called a physician in search for the etiological factor. This physician happened to be reading my thesis and let him have it, with the result of the article which I have enclosed.

The physician advised against mentioning my name because it would be publicity, etc. But I feel content in my own mind that a job is well done. That is more important to me. But you can imagine how surprised I was when I read the paper & found the quotations & recognized them from my thesis, which I thought was safely in the library.

And again—all of my love to you.

Joe

NEW ORLEANS
Thurs. Nite, April 28

Dearest Joe—

Only 40 more days and our state board exams should be over, and all I'm looking forward to is seeing you and your folks soon afterward. Every time anyone mentions our month of vacation, I'm sure my face takes on such a beam that people must think I am slightly "tetched"—I wonder if I am.

We are excused from a few classes next week to attend the State Medical Convention meetings. However, I'm afraid I'll gain more information by staying home and digging. I haven't decided how much of the weekend that includes—I'll hate to miss my usual afternoon show on Sundays!

However, Dr. H.O. Barker from Alexandria may come down and if he does, we'll probably have a little conference. He's a former Veterans Bureau doctor, but quit the service a few years ago and is now chief of the only hospital in Alex, the Baptist hospital. He may have quite some competition now that the state is building a Charity Hospital in Pineville.

The seniors are urged to attend a faculty club meeting tomorrow night—which means one less night to study. However, I'm curious to attend one of these.

Dot joins me in a "Goodnight" to you.

Love,
Alice

Omaha
Monday, May 2
2:30

Darling:

Pediatrics dispensary is over soon, so now I am sitting in the card room at the house waiting for the mailman. And to the tune of Bing Crosby in "Palace in Paradise," what could be more appropriate than to write to you. Could we call Rochester our palace in Paradise—six weeks of perfect companionship—and now we both sailed away. Any place would be paradise with you. Now, I'll play "Dancing Under the Stars," also by Bing. Wouldn't it be perfect if we could do that tonight? Yes, I am quite a dreamer—but, gee, it's fun. I hope that you share my dreams. Now let us have some swing numbers—perhaps "Sophisticated Swing"?

It is warm enough for my gray suit today—practically summer.

As I look around the card room I see pictures of Nu Sigma Nu alumni. There is Dr. Will Mayo, Dr. Earl Sage, head of OB & Gyn—and he does not have a flower in his lapel. How did that ever happen? Perhaps the photographer caught him too early in the morning. And Dr. George Prichard still has his mustache—but now it is gray. And Dr. Charles Rex Kennedy without a cigarette. Gee, they are a grand group of physicians—every one of them. I hope that someday my students & patients, if any, will think one-tenth as much of me as we think of them. Therefore we must try to follow the standards that they set up.

And the card table—what stories it could tell—evenings of poker, cribbage, and bridge. It could tell tales of men now quite prominent in medicine. I wonder who burned that cigarette hole in it.

Now more music. "My First Impression of You."

Where is the mailman or is this a holiday?

Nola is scheduled for another shower at 4 this afternoon.

2:55

Time for class—and I hope the mailman is coming up Farnam Street so I can meet him.

8:30

Darling—

Nola got a bath and I took quite a shower doing it. And now she is more beautiful than ever.

Above all, I received your letter.

Went to the Methodist Hospital to see a patient from the Home. After that, Nola & I rode around listening to the Lux Radio Theatre. Gary Cooper in "The Prisoner of Shark Island."

What a candid shot subject I would make now. It is very hot— and there is one way to cool if without a fan, & that is to remove tie, collar, shirt & shoes.

About the vacation—my plans are going sky high. I am afraid two weeks will be too short. But we will make the best of it. Now let's hope and pray that everything will turn out OK so that we can go.

Goodnight to Dot and for you, my love.

Joe

OMAHA
Monday, May 9
10:15

Dearest Alice:

What a weekend. This makes ten rush weeks that I have been active in (6 spring & 4 fall rush weeks), and this was the most fatiguing. Thursday night the fellows started coming in. Friday we took them to class and had an entertainment & smokes at the house for them in the evening. We showed some of Mead Johnson & Co.'s medical pictures, and did the rushees go for that. Later it developed into a beer party with crap games & jokes, but I managed to steer clear of both. We put up fourteen beds in the dorm last week, and they were all full. It seemed that everyone decided to leave their clothes in our room. I tried on several pairs of shoes before I found mine.

Saturday the pre-meds were guests of the University Hospital, & we had to act as guides to take them through the buildings & to the clinics. In the afternoon we had our clinic at the house. Dr. Ralph Luikart, one of our alumni from Penn. & from the dept. of OB at Creighton, put on an OB demonstration. He brought his manikin & a pickled fetus and showed everything from a normal left occiput anterior position to a complicated abdominal presentation. Frankly, I learned a lot of OB. Dr. Luikart also developed a modification of the Keilland, Tucker-McLane & Simpson forceps, which has the fetal side fenestrated & pelvic side smooth.

And the party Saturday night—the continuous rain of Friday & Saturday turned to sleet & snow Saturday night. It melted soon but did spoil the party a little. We had a nice crowd, but I only wish that you had been there. Some of the rushees drank a little, but on the whole it was quite a sober party & very respectable.

Sunday was a clear cool day and I went home. Nola made the trip in 2 hours. It was certainly quite a pleasure to be home on Mother's

Day. Our home is being remodeled & Mother has changed the arrangement of the kitchen almost completely.

Four weeks from today and graduation. Is it possible?

Love,

Joe

NEW ORLEANS
Early Thurs. a.m., May 12

Dearest Joe—

The time that I've been cramming has really been all too short, but I was so unused to studying that it seems ages since I've done anything else. Well, just 1 week and 2 days more and it will be all over—I hope. At any rate, there are supposed to be no repeaters next year and I'll be out, one way or another, either on my ear or on my feet with a sheepskin.

Rush week must be a combination of pleasure and hard work. That's one thing we medico-eds don't have to worry about. We have no competition, and as yet have had no girl in school who didn't desire to join AEI. Quite a saving, isn't it! By the way, I hear that the only two other medical fraternities for women take in associate professions such as veterinarians, osteopaths, chiropodists, etc. Which makes me prouder than ever of AEI.

We have been told of Dr. Luikart's forceps—and given favorable reports on it. It must have been a rare privilege to get to hear him speak—and particularly, see the mannikin demonstrations.

Mother writes me that Dad caught about 50 fish last weekend and that friends came over for a big fish fry. The strawberry shortcake, whipped cream, coffee, etc., surely made my mouth water. I hope we can have a similar one sometime during June.

Your graduation is one week later than ours. How I wish we could attend both. Gee, I can hardly wait for the middle of June to come. Sometimes I get to dreaming about you so much that I almost catch myself speaking aloud to your picture—and our Psychiatry course teaches that that is a bad sign! Guess I'm hopeless.

Hope you can read this—I doubt if even I could.

Love,
Alice

OMAHA
Thursday, May 12

Dearest:

Just try to get any studying done around here. First it was about five juniors in here studying Gyn for their examination tonight. Later, one by one the freshmen came in, perhaps to borrow some paper, get a book, read a magazine or just talk. One of our freshmen is very depressed tonight—and for a very good reason. The anatomy professor practically told him that he will flunk. He is a very studious fellow—he studies more than any other freshman—but it seems that he has been a "marked man" since school started. For months they have tried to force him to quit, but he is too stubborn. He would make a swell doctor. He has a pleasing personality, is an interesting & witty conversationalist and has other qualities of a good doctor. For four years I have seen men forced out of school— good fellows—and it makes me wonder whether the work that a man does in his freshman year is a good criterion as to whether he will make a good physician or not.

Our examinations last the 18th–24th. Comprehensives the 27th. Just something to worry about.

Now Keith Krausnick decided to tell some stories about his ranch out west. What a place this is getting to be. Perhaps it is because it is so close to school.

Harry Powers & Vincent Swanson are going to intern at Ancher Hospital at St. Paul next year. I wonder where the rest of the summer group will be. I hope someday that we get to meet them at Mayo's.

23 more days—how short it will seem.

Now Keith is branding cattle & riding broncos on his ranch. What a storyteller.

Until Monday.

> Love,
> Joe

> Omaha
> Sunday afternoon, May 15
> 3:35

Darling:

I feel a little depressed and this is the best way to pep up my spirits. Today we had a Mother's Day dinner at the house, and wives & sweethearts of Nu Sigs were also present. My mother found it impossible to come because they had some church festival and she was in charge of one of the committees. That was quite a disappointment, and your being 1,200 miles away did not help much. I wish that both of you could have been here. A.C. went to Lincoln yesterday and has not returned and I don't blame him, since he has been an orphan for 15 years. Perhaps that is why we are so much like brothers, because my parents have tried to take their place. Whenever Mother made me a scarf, sweater, etc., she made one for A.C., too. It will be tough to separate on graduation.

I see that the Czechoslovak crisis is becoming rather grave. No doubt you know where I stand in that. Why don't they let the peaceful Czechs alone—they never hurt anyone. But the greed for power sees no boundaries.

Examinations this week. It is too nice to study indoors, and if you would be here I know just the place to go. Out, away from anyone, under the shade of a tree. No doubt we would not study but rather pick flowers, walk around the lake or listen to the birds. But today Nola and I will go there together, & undoubtedly I will look up from the pages many times & dream that you would be sitting beside me.

I saved some flowers from the dinner table and now they are beside your picture.

Love,
Joe

NEW ORLEANS
Wed. Afternoon, May 18

Dearest Joe—

My folks are getting more excited even than I about graduation and are insisting on giving me new clothes, etc., although I've told them not to, because I'll be in white all next year. I just hope everything goes off fine for their sake, too. People are just too good to me and I know I don't deserve it—and I am not fishing.

Well, we're half through our exams. Medicine and Surgery are over—and now our chief worries are Pediatrics, Neuropsychiatry, and Orthopedics.

I suppose you are in the midst of exams now. I wish the best for you, and I know you'll finish everything in the very proficient way characterizing all your actions.

I know you'll overlook the shortness of the letter, and I'd better prepare you for a long one as soon as exams are over.

Love,
Alice

Omaha

Friday, May 20

Darling:

Everything has happened during the last week. We are in the midst of about a dozen things.

First, examinations. Had two in medicine and one in orthopedics today. Surgery Monday, tropical medicine Tuesday. On Thursday comes the big comprehensive, and we can expect anything. It has been a rule to give only one subject and to write 3 hours on it. Here are some of the subjects:

Fever	1935
Edema	1936
Anemia	1937

This includes discussing all of the embryology, anatomy, path, physiology, bio-chem, pharmacology, diseases and treatment of the conditions. Cerebral spinal fluid, dyspepsia, jaundice would be good questions this year. I believe that I could write all that I know about these in 15 minutes.

Some of the staff are having dinners & parties for the seniors. Dr. C.C. Tomlinson, chairman of Dermatology, is having a dinner next Wed. and, of course, we must attend the Dean's tea the 29th. State boards are June 8th. Several of the alumni were here this week. Dr. Raymond Joseph Wyrens, who had Dr. Mac's fellowship in 1934, has had 3 years of medicine in the East & now wants to start practicing, and apparently it is very hard to get located.

And thanks for the lovely graduation announcement. I have been parading all over the house with it. I only wish that I could be there the 30th. I see that our former bishop, the Most Reverend Joseph Rummel, will give the Baccalaureate Sermon.

I am still waiting for an OB to deliver to whom I gave 3 grains of luminal last Friday. One week overdue already. Induction should be indicated soon. This is keeping me with my arm around a telephone expecting the call anytime.

And now a goodnight kiss for you.

Love,
Joe

NEW ORLEANS
Saturday, May 21

Dearest Joe—

What a grand time. Exams are all over, and I'm still keeping my fingers crossed until I hear from them. I heard all the class passed surgery, and I made the second highest grade in medicine—will you excuse the boasting, but I am proud of it. I'm still hoping that the school will have to break its record of failing seniors and pass everyone in our class. I hear they received a letter from the AMA this year about failing seniors. It does seem that it should be unnecessary. There is no one in our class doing outstanding work, one way or another. We're all on a pretty even keel, and I don't see how they could fail any of us.

I thought of you specially when studying a lecture in Preventive Medicine on Ventilation. A temperature above 60°F makes one more susceptible to upper respiratory infection, disinclined to exertion, causes a rise in body temperature and a decrease in the efficiency of our vasomotor control. And here it was 88° here yesterday and 90° today. One nice thing, it didn't start getting so warm until just about 3 days ago, and the weather was very comfortable during most of our period of study.

I'm very anxious for you to make a personal study on the climatic conditions down here, especially in Alex and N.O. I hope you don't find it too unpleasant.

Ah, how I hope we soon find out the final results. I'm hoping that we hear Monday so I can go home that day or the next.

I phoned Mother last night to tell her my work was all over, and she said yes, that she too had been counting the days. I really believe my folks are getting as much pleasure out of this as I am, and they certainly deserve to. I wish so much that I could do something to really show them that I appreciate them.

I'll be earning all of $10 a month next year (I hope). Can't I do lots with that!

Dot and I went shopping this afternoon after I finally got up. I had threatened to sleep until 7 p.m. but had to get to school for 1 p.m. to check out of Medicine Lab. We found some very nice—and reasonable—white tailored and sanforized suits, so we ordered enough to complete our supply of intern suits. I'm hoping that will take a load off Mother's shoulders. Oh, yes, I expect to be in Alex next Thursday—remember, it's 1733 White St.—but will probably be in N.O. during the next week as State Boards come June 2, 3, and 4. But this week will probably be filled with your exams, and I will understand if you don't find time to write so often. I'll miss the letters terribly, but I don't ever want to cause you the slightest bit of trouble. Would I could find some way to help you and give you just a bit of the inspiration you have given me, Dr. Holoubek!!

Love,
Alice

OMAHA

Sunday, May 29

Dearest Alice:

I have some good news to tell you—I passed. Surprised? Not half as much as I am. All of the examinations are over and only 4 fellows flunked the comprehensives. These got another chance at the "Bed-sides"—they are each given a patient, and 4–5 staff men fire questions at them for some time until the student is practically exhausted. None have flunked the last four years, and I am certain that the men will get through OK this year.

The three-hour question was Friday. "Acute Abdomen." Books have been written on that subject, but to organize & outline the material so that it could be written in 3 hours was some task. Think of all of the possibilities, dozens of them. But all I know is that I passed—I still cannot believe it. Now 2 more days of Pediatrics dispensary & I am through. Lab is over, thank goodness.

Last Wed. p.m. the orders were to quit studying and go to Dr. Tomlinson's country home. We played softball for hours—yes, there were more errors than hits. My hands still hurt—I played first base without a glove.

Took some photos—hope they come out. After dinner each fellow had to do some form of entertainment. What a floor show. Four of us Bohemians sang songs, another chap auctioned off everything in the house. And you should have heard one fellow mimicking our instructors—it was a scream. The best part came when one of the fellows asked Dr. Tomlinson, "How can a fellow practice honest medicine and own such a grand place as this?" The answer was, "It's the skin game."

And then we gave the Dean a loaded cigarette and I had Argus focused for the picture—but the load never went off. Rats.

The party was over at 9:30—and nothing to drink but coffee & water. Which proved that meds can have a good time without intoxicants.

The Dean is having a tea for us in about—no, it started 15 minutes ago—well, I'll be late.

How I wish I could be at your graduation. Congratulations—a million times. I hope to deliver them in person someday.

But now, just pretend that I am there—and from now on it will be Dr. Alice Baker. How does it feel to be actually through? I should know in one week. I hope.

The fellows are gathering in the room, so I had better get Nola & we will be off to the Dean's. I plan to go home for Memorial Day & return Tuesday—

> Love,
> Joe

Good luck on the state boards, but I know that you will pass them easily.

NEW ORLEANS
Tues nite, May 31

Dearest Joe—

What a grand time I have had. The only thing lacking is that which I have known only since meeting you. You were missed so very much. With each event was the feeling—if Joe were only here with me. I was so glad to get back to 116 So. Johnson where I knew a letter would be waiting. And what did I find—not only a letter, always so welcome and enjoyed, but a graduation announcement and the loveliest gift. You are undoubtedly the most thoughtful person I've ever known.

I am so delighted with my folks. You should hear them talk about you. I really believe they think they are looking forward to you and your parents' visit as much as I am, but I know that isn't possible. Oh, how great it will be to see you.

Your announcement is lovely. And those university buildings just seem to be inspiring—don't they add an incentive to one's drive to learn? And is the university hospital the one in Omaha or is it the one connected to the Lincoln campus?

We had a very lovely graduation. As you saw, there were almost 1,000 students to receive degrees, so instead of having the exercises in the Greek amphitheatre as usual, it was necessary to hold them in the stadium. I was surprised, but a lovely setting was provided and the nights were cool and clear, for which we were thankful.

Yes, for the first time in the history of the school I believe, every senior med student passed. And were we proud to march up on that platform and get our diplomas. I had asked my folks to sit near the aisle down which we marched, and as I spoke to them in passing I heard my Dad say, "That is my baby"—and it's one time I didn't fuss with him over it. Goodness knows he and Mother deserve that diploma more than I do. I was so happy that they were feeling fine again and could come.

As for being surprised that you passed—why, it's absurd. My dear, you with your fine ideals, wonderful mind, and perseverance typify a true physician—and I'm sure you've heard enough from me on that subject to know what I mean.

I've been looking forward to your visit with great anticipation, but as June approaches, the yearning grows greater.

My love,
Alice

OMAHA
Friday night, June 3

Dearest:

What a night—went to see "Cocoanut Grove" with one of the freshmen (or I should say sophomores now). After that, to the Port Bar, and
over a glass of beer we discussed everything from medicine to philosophy. Later, back to the house, and four more fellows anxious to voice
their opinions about school, instructors, and medicine in general.

One more hour of dispensary—my, what a relief—and Monday is
graduation. What an eventful day. There were times that we felt that it
would never come. Now we can count the hours instead of the days.

Your parents are justly proud of you—and why shouldn't they be.
It is so rare an achievement for a young lady, particularly to finish
so high in her class. And I am proud of you too.

A.C. is making plans to leave for Rochester during the middle
of June. Don't we envy him—but we should have a very enjoyable
summer if only a fraction of the time is available.

I plan to go home the 9th of June, and we should leave the 12th.

Nola is in perfect shape. She has a scratch on the underside of one
fender and even though it does not show, it still breaks my heart.

The pen is perfect. I know it will last a lifetime and it will always
be a reminder of you.

Love,

Joe

CLARKSON
Friday night, June 10

Dearest Alice:

This week certainly has been filled with activity—not even a minute to sit down and relax. Perhaps it is the climate.

I went to Lincoln Sunday afternoon. What a dead town compared to Omaha. Only recently the Blue Law was repealed and they started having shows on Sundays.

Commencement Monday—I managed to keep awake during the speeches—and what a thrill to finally get the diploma. After all of these years. What a memorable day. Father, Mother and my sister & her husband were down. It was certainly quite a thrill for my folks. Gee, I hope that someday I can repay them for all that they have done for me.

After graduation I tried to spend Tuesday studying for state boards, but it was very difficult. Somehow or other the old ambition left me. Nevertheless, I did manage to scan through my Therapeutics book.

The questions could have been easier. Medicine and pharmacology were the most difficult, surgery, the easiest. As far as I have heard, no one has flunked the boards for 8 years, but, of course, there is always a chance. I can rest in peace for one month because it will take that long to grade them.

What fun I had packing. Part of my books & clothes were left behind, and I will take them directly to the hospital.

I arrived home this morning. A.C. was here for dinner and we certainly enjoyed going through my high school photographs. Four out of 36 are married.

Our intern's uniforms came Wednesday. $25.00 for 6 suits—yes, pleated backs and everything, but no gold buttons.

My parents certainly appreciate the kind invitation of your father and mother and, of course, it is settled, we will come. However, we have to spend a day in Kansas City and so may not get there until the 16th. I will wire you a day ahead.

Gee, but I am anxious to see you & your folks and to talk old times over again. And as far as doing things with you—anything that you plan as long as you are along. But there should be a dance sometime. Imagine, a week from now & I will be with you.

Until, then, my love, and I'll wire you the 15th or 16th.

Love,

Joe

'One week was not enough'

June 1938

Darling Alice:

I miss you so much tonight. If I could only hold you in my arms for a little while—or just hold your hand once more. Why didn't we make it 1 hour longer last night? I'll continue to see your face before me always, but I would like to look at you now like I did last night. That was perfect.

For one week we have been together almost all of the time and always under the same roof—and today 530 miles away, and tomorrow 400 more. Yes, it is very difficult to take.

The hardest thing that I have ever done was to leave Alexandria today & to leave you behind. And I almost turned back—now I wish I had. And it was hard driving through the tears.

Mother forgot her camera and some plants behind but I left something more important—you.

I almost forgot to tell you about the trip. Nola works perfectly—and a story to tell on my dad. He said, "This is the way to drive—50 miles an hour, like Alice," but later I saw the speedometer creep up to 75, so I guess it's in our blood—but I promise to go slowly tomorrow.

And the lunch that your mother fixed was grand—thanks a million. I think she is very, very nice. I didn't have time to thank her for everything but do it for me, please.

Sorry, dear, but I am very tired today and will write a longer letter when I get home.

Love,
Joe

ALEXANDRIA
Wed. Night, June 22

My dearest Joe—

I suppose that by now you are almost to Oklahoma City. I do hope you could sleep today and haven't been too awfully tired.

I've missed you so very, very much today—but yet, I still seem so filled with the happiness of having you here that I suppose it is nothing to how I will miss you. But I do know I wish Nola were in front and we could find some excuse—as if the folks were ever fooled—to leave in it together. Thank goodness, it won't be long until work starts and I have lots to do until then. Mother hasn't quite finished my intern suits, and I have a couple of pairs of pajamas, etc., to make.

I got to read just a few pages of the thesis this afternoon. And Joe, it is so interesting. I knew I would enjoy it, just knowing that you had written it, but my goodness, I had no idea it would be that interesting. Do you know—that ought to be published in book form. If it can settle the question of climate and disease, every student and doctor should have it. But it is more than a collection of facts—at least, so I gathered from talking to you—and so interesting I think everyone should read it.

Of course, I haven't gotten to those parts about the South yet. Maybe I'll change my mind—Ha. No, I'll remember you wrote that before you came to the "Sunny South."

I can't think of any news to tell you. All I can do is send you my love again and again—and tell you how I love your parents too. Oh, I'm so, so happy you could come.

> My love,
> Alice

CLARKSON
Thursday Night, June 23

Sweetheart:

We just got unpacked—what a mess.

Gee, can it be that a little over 48 hours ago you & I were dancing to "Harbor Lights"? And then we listened to Freddie Ebner's orchestra from Omaha and talked for over an hour. But it seemed much too short. Could we only turn time backward—or rather, forward—a year. I love you.

We had quite a trip home from Lincoln. Due to the heavy rains west of here, the Platte River was over its banks south of Schuyler & the roads had from 2–3 feet of water on it. Nola said, "I think I can, I think I can." And we went fine. Then, about the time that we had 3 inches of water above the floor boards in the seat, Nola said, "I'm drowning"—and she did. Well, a State Highway truck pushed us the remainder of the way, and after a few coughs, Nola started again. It was quite a sight to see. Nola plowing through the water and half the fender submerged.

Yes, we had a few rains here & the lawn has grown by feet. The roses have opened and they are beautiful—but not half as nice as the flowers & trees in Alexandria.

Gee, I feel low tonight, but as soon as I start that internship—well, I may be kept busier, but that still won't prevent me from thinking of you. Let us hope that it will only be a year.

Again, I am rather tired & will write more tomorrow.

With all my love,

Joe

ALEXANDRIA

Thurs. nite, June 23

My dearest—

I was so very glad to get that telegram. I was hoping so for one and so glad it came early. You must have made excellent time. How were the roads—and was it very hot and dry?

Mother and I guess that you are at your sister's tonight. I'll bet she is glad you are back—but not half as glad as we are sorry! I'm already looking forward to a return visit.

You should see Mother and me reading your thesis. We have a time, both of us reading at once, but manage it pretty well. I can't get over how interesting you've made it. And I do hope I may take it to the Hospital with me for I know Dot wants to read it. I also want to take your advice and read some more on the history of medicine and the "Works of Hippocrates."

Oh, how much I miss you. And the radio is such a sweet reminder. I find it awfully hard to keep my mind upon any subject excepting you. I'm looking forward to my Thursday letter just a day late this time.

All my love, dear,

Alice

CLARKSON
Friday night, June 24

Darling:

Just took A.C. home after he spent the evening here. Your ears should be ringing continuously because I have been talking about you constantly. Even about the dresses you wear & the way your hair is fixed. I like everything about you.

A.C. finally asked, "When is she coming down? I want to meet her." Shall we give him his wish? But be careful, he is a good looking, black curly-haired chap.

Everyone wants to know what impressed us the most on our trip south. Darling, there is only one answer. It is you. In fact, I only remember the places where we were together. The Arkansas Ozarks have no place in my memory. But that certain spot on Pontchartrain Beach Drive does. And even the mosquitoes of Louisiana are nice.

And I like Mother & Daddy Baker very much. The preserves were delicious. It was a rare treat to taste them. The French coffee & Evangeline sauce are being saved for Sunday when my sister, Louis & Dennis & A.C. will come over. Your mother certainly picked out the things that I liked best (yes, and even the hot stuff). And the cotton bale is just what I wanted. Thank her for me, please. I still want to go on the fishing trip with your father. It would be grand sport, especially with him.

Darling, I like all of your friends so much. The Tysons & John Charles, Dot, Bernes, Aunty & especially Dr. Will O'D. Jones. They are all so very nice. And I am sorry that I could not meet your other friends, but I assure you we will the next time.

We went to Adela's today, and Dennis is just as lively as ever, even though he is cutting a new tooth. And what a smile. So much like John Charles. Oh, you must meet him sometime.

Apparently you have not read the most radical part of my thesis yet. And please do not change your mind about me after that. Much of it seems like a flight of ideas. But the problem of climate is not settled yet, as you will see. All I did was lay a foundation—I hope.

I miss you, sweetheart, but we must stand it another year even though it will be more difficult. And then, well, we hope & pray that our dreams will come true. I love you & will kiss you in my dreams. I will go to Omaha Thursday.

Joe

CLARKSON
Saturday, June 25

My Dearest Alice:

It has turned very cool here—in fact, several blankets are very desirable. Changeable Nebraska weather.

Sweetheart—only one week ago we saw some of the night life of N.O. and we danced to "Harbor Lights." Those memories will never die with me. I wish that we could go out for a poor boy sandwich now. Mother wants Clotile here to help her, but the only time anyone dares have a maid here is when they are ill. Such funny customs these northerners, especially Clarksonians, have.

A.C. is leaving for Rochester Monday. I hope that we can go up there together for a few days in September and for sure for 3 years in September of 1939. Wouldn't that be perfect?

There are so many things that I had wanted to tell you, but one week was not enough. My parents send their love and regards and wish to thank you & your father and mother for the hospitality extended to us. That made it the most pleasant trip that we have ever taken, and we hope that we can repay it whenever you come to Nebraska. And please, dear, if you drive up, take three days for the trip—fast driving is not safe in any car, even Nola or Happy.

I love you more & more.

Joe

Alexandria
Saturday, June 25

Dearest Joe—

Good ole Nola—it takes a real car to start after having been drowned by such a deluge. The rain seems to be haunting you on this trip, doesn't it?

Oh! I wish the trip were just starting instead of just having ended, and I could have that perfect week to live over again. Oh, my dear, how I do miss you! I've been going to bed at the earliest hour in years. It would be too lonely to stay up now by myself as I had been doing. And surprisingly enough, the early morning hours are very pleasant, and one can get much more done.

Yesterday our preacher talked on Christian love, and his text was the beautiful thirteenth chapter of First Corinthians. I've never heard a more beautiful sermon. Then, although I was with old friends all day, I spent the whole day with you. You especially liked the gardenias we picked, did you not? They were very pretty in spite of being the latest ones of the season.

And guess what Dad brought me the other day. He has a very valued friend, Father L.A. DuPont, priest of the Pineville Catholic Church, and they have long talks about religion. So the Father loaned Dad a book—"Plain Reasons for Being a Catholic" by Rev. Albert Power. I've read only the first chapter as yet but find it very interesting. I hope I get to finish it before I go back to N.O.

You should see all our figs—we get about 4 gallons every day, or every other day, at least. So we are going to have some good preserves. I think they're even better than the fresh fig, don't you?

My dear, I love you. I've never said that to anyone else and don't intend to. I'm hoping that interning keeps me so busy I won't have too much time to think and to miss you, although I would be lost if I couldn't think of you—oh, you know what I mean—and a year isn't forever, and we have lots to look forward to. Give my love to your folks—it is yours anyway—

Alice

CLARKSON
Sunday, June 26

My Darling:

Don Ameche is just singing "I Fall in Love With You Every Day."
And I do hope that you are listening too, dear.

Adela thanks you very much for the booklet on New Orleans
that you sent her. And, of course, she is very, very anxious to meet
you. Dennis is as active as ever. And we had French coffee, canned
figs and other dishes from the cookbook. The preserves that your
mother sent are going too fast—everyone likes them.

I plan to send this letter to Alexandria yet & I hope that you will
still be there. My address will be University Hospital, 42nd & Dewey
Ave., after next Thursday.

Later

A.C. is leaving for Omaha tomorrow & Rochester on Tuesday. Yes,
I told him the important things, especially to look up Mary Lomasney & also to put in a good word for Dr. Baker & Dr. Holoubek
whenever possible.

Until the next letter—I love you with all my heart.

Joe

ALEXANDRIA
Tues. a.m., June 28

Dearest—

The time is coming! Do you have the slight dread of the first weeks of internship that I do? I feel so very inadequate, but I know very well I'll enjoy it thoroughly after I get started. Anyway it won't be long now. I suppose I'll have to leave tomorrow. And thank goodness it will make the time pass more quickly.

I think it is a good thing I didn't find time to read your thesis too rapidly for it might have gotten me. As it was, only two or three statements really bothered me. I'll have you know, sir, that it's an insult to say a Southerner is lacking in courage—and it will probably call for a fight at once. I can't correlate it with the climate, but I do know that Southerners are hot-headed as the dickens. Of course, the intelligence part—well, Mother says the northerners don't recognize our heroes as great men. But I would really feel sorry for you if you read parts of that thesis before a Southern Medical Convention.

And doggone it, it's such a darned good thesis, and so very interesting! I knew it had taken a lot of work, but I didn't appreciate half how much. Really, you are certainly a most interesting writer. I've never heard you speak in public, but with such a facility of expressing yourself in such an interesting way, and with the practice that presidency in such a large frat chapter must mean, I'll bet there is little room for improvement. I'm so very proud of you.

I'm expecting Dr. Jones over to eat more fish with us tonight—Dad caught quite a few yesterday—and I hope he'll get started on Mayo's. And oh, how I wish you were to be here again. I know I'll think of each of you with each bite of fish.

All my love to you—
Alice

CLARKSON
Tuesday, June 28
9 p.m.

My dearest Alice:

Again we spent an evening talking about the South and what a perfectly lovely time we had at your home.

One more evening to spend at home and then for a year's solid work. But don't worry, dear, I will not work too hard. And everything that I do will be for you.

I believe that you are leaving for Charity tomorrow. I do hope that they have better quarters for you than the two rooms that you mentioned. And please, dear, do be careful, especially when you are on accident service—and also, please stay as far from the TB patients as possible. I do not know what I would do if you should get sick. Perhaps take the next train south.

Yes, I am doing well in catching up on my rest—sleep from 9 to 8. It couldn't be sleeping sickness.

I spent about 3 hours talking to one of the Clarkson physicians today. He thoroughly discouraged Clarkson as a place to practice & recommended Iowa or Indiana. However, I prefer the South, and it isn't only because I like the climate.

And I do love the Louisiana moon. Will it be full the next time that we see it together?

With all my love & oh how I miss you.

Joe

NEW ORLEANS
Wed. Nite, June 29

Dearest—

Well, it's New Orleans again. And even though I do hate to leave home, I'm always glad to return. Old Canal Street surely has a charm of its own.

Your letter was so nice. Mother appreciated your thanks, and I know enjoyed so much getting the different things for you. Do you know, I've never heard my folks be so wholehearted in their approval and liking of anyone before, especially in such a short time. Goodness knows I am glad—and can understand it perfectly.

Dr. Jones came over last night, and you should have heard him. First he said, "Alice, I like your boyfriend. He seems very nice." Then he started quizzing me—asking me what you wanted to specialize in, what you planned to do when you finished your internship, where you intended to practice, etc. He ended by saying that he didn't want to seem inquisitive but he did want to know—and that was the only way he could find out. Then he started talking about Mayo's, etc., and urged me to write for an application as soon as possible.

Well, Dot had taken care of everything—she selected our room here, and had everything lined up—and Bernes and I had a grand time talking. She and Dot rave about you so much I almost get jealous, but I do enjoy talking about you so much, and it's so nice for them to know you too, so they'll know I don't exaggerate.

Dot's trying to sleep. I'll have lots to write tomorrow nite so for now—good night, dear, and all my love,

Alice

OMAHA
Wed. night, June 29
9:10

My darling Alice:

Dearest, I wish that you would be here tonight. I miss you more everyday. But now my hospital duties may keep me busy part of the day. However, there are three very important parts to my day—morning at 10 I receive your letter, 7 p.m. to write to you, and after 10 to dream of you.

I came to Omaha about 4:30 today and am moved into my room. It is a single, about 7'x12', with a window on the west & door on the east. A single bed in the northwest corner, book shelf & desk in southwest, dresser along south wall & a 2½'x3'x8' metal locker in the southeast corner. Mother made a nice padded cover for my trunk, so that is along the south wall too.

And the two things that I am most proud of—your picture on the dresser & the LSU tiger on my desk.

Incidentally, I am on anesthetics—a very easy service to start on but very confining because I have to be present at all OBs.

Received your Monday letter just before I left home, and what a thrill it was to read it. I have some very good friends among the priests, too, and talks with them are very inspiring. I would like to meet Father DuPont sometime.

Nola's voice (her horn) was rather hoarse this week, and only yesterday it finally all dried out after that drowning it received.

Would I like to be picking figs with you, dearest.

Let us hope that this next year passes very, very rapidly, sweetheart. And you know that I love you with all of my heart and am thinking of you constantly.

My love always,
Joe

NEW ORLEANS
Thurs. Nite, June 30

Dearest one—

My, I've been called Dr. so often today that I'll bet my head has enlarged. However, I know it will be shrunk tomorrow, probably to less than normal size. I do dread tomorrow fiercely, but guess I'll live over it.

I'm assigned to Dibert Tuberculosis Hospital on my first service, along with white male medicine and dermatology. I'll be glad to get it off my hands first. Oh, yes, and my tick call is 3-3-2. It's been running through my head ever since they told me, but I'm sure I'll never hear it when it's for me.

I saw Gamble tonight. He's just the same, and I told him you had been down. He had bad luck in the room proposition. We are having more interns and residents this year than ever before. Consequently, the intern quarters are very crowded. So to make room, the hospital is renting a small frame building back of the ambulance house. Until the building is ready for occupancy, the interns are living 3–4 to a room.

But the girls have it nice. The residents have their old rooms in the convalescent building, 6th floor, and we interns are located on the first floor of Milliken, which also contains the dining room (basement) and white pediatrics, OB, and observation room.

Dot and I have the only double room and the only room with two windows. We also, thank goodness, have a large electric fan. But the current must be D.C. instead of A.C. for my little fan from home won't run, and my radio started fizzing and burning when I plugged it in. However, I think we can remedy that. I surely hope so for I missed Bing tonight.

I'll ask very soon if I can apply now for a week's vacation in September—but there I go hoping and wishing again. But now I have much more faith in my dreams coming true.

Goodnight, dear, and my love to you—

Alice

TWO

❧

INTERNSHIP
Nebraska & Louisiana

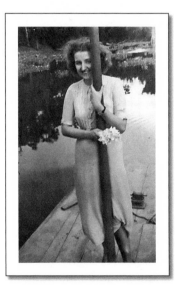

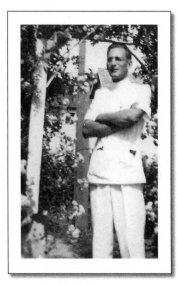

Dr. Alice Baker, June 1938,
boating on Bayou Teche in
southern Louisiana

Dr. Joe Holoubek, June 1938,
family rose garden, Clarkson,
Nebraska

'About Rochester . . .'

⟹⊷●⊷⟸

OMAHA
Thurs. night, June 30
7:40

My darling Alice:

I just came up from OB where I gave an anesthetic. I started to work officially at 5:30 tonight and have been quite busy ever since. Our regular anesthetist is in California on a vacation, and the former intern on the service will leave on Saturday, so after that, heaven help the patients, because I will be the only one left. Imagine, me with ether, nitrous oxide, cyclopropane & avertin to give. I hope they don't ask for evipal. That will keep my mornings busy, & in the p.m. I have to dictate letters to the M.D.'s who sent in the patients. That involves summarizing the hospital charts, etc.—more fun. And I am constantly on call for OBs & emergencies.

I am telling everyone from the janitor to the Dean about my trip south and about you, dear. I started with the Dean yesterday, and we spent a very pleasant half hour discussing the south & N.O. & LSU. Finally, when we mentioned Mayo's, "You have my permission to apply," he said. We write to Donald C. Balfour, M.D., Director, University of Minnesota Graduate School, the Mayo Foundation, Rochester. And he said that Dr. Wilder is the big gun on the Committee. Darling, we must have him pull for us.

And guess what I did today—called all bus & railroad stations.

BUS Round Trip $26.30
Leave Alex   3:45 p.m.
Arrive Omaha   11:05 p.m.—next day
Leave Omaha   7:45 a.m.
Arrive Alex   9:10 P.M—next day

TRAIN Round Trip to Alex $33.55
Leave Omaha   11:59 p.m.
Arrive Alex   10:10 a.m.—next day

AIR Round Trip to N.O. $97
Leave Omaha   7:45 p.m.
Arrive N.O.   3:33 a.m.—next day
Leave N.O.   1:15 p.m.
Arrive Omaha   11:29 p.m.—same day

Imagine, I am only 7 hours & 48 minutes away from you. Well, someday—perhaps.

I read the 13th chapter of Corinthians—it is very, very beautiful. One chapter from the Bible every night for me.

> Darling, I love you dearly,
> Joe

OMAHA
Friday, July 1
4:45

My adorable one:

My first ether case was a tonsillectomy, & hot dog was I scared. But so far none died, although a spinal anesthesia case dropped blood pressure from 140/70 to 70/50 in about a minute, but adrenalin brought her out of it.

And what a job to dictate the letters. It necessitates reviewing the charts & only mentioning the essentials. It is a new experience but very valuable. But I dread the 5th when we will have all of the dismissals of 2, 3 & 4.

Received my schedule today:

July	Anesthetics
August	Admitting room & nose & throat
September	OB
October	Gyn
November	Pediatrics & Oral Surgery
December	Neurology & Ophthalmology
January	Orthopedics & Urology
February	Radiology & Dermatology
March/April	Medicine
May/June	Surgery

So you see, I can go to Rochester in Sept. & the remainder of the vacation in Dec. or Jan. or Feb. What is your schedule, darling? Mine starts very easy but will end with the two heaviest services.

Dear, I've been telling everyone about you & the South. Yes, I even got into several good arguments when I stood up for Huey Long.

Darling, I love you and only you. And another year of being apart won't be forever.

I'm thinking of you always.

Love,

Joe

NEW ORLEANS

Fri. Nite, July 1

Dearest—

What a day! Am I tired! And so on, far into the night. Oh, and talk about surprise. I was over a patient's bed with another resident, Dr. David Fader, when Dr. J.O. Weilbaecher walked up. He's Chief of the Medical Service and as nice as can be. All of a sudden he pointed to my Nu Sigma Nu pin and said, "Where did you get that?" It surprised me so I could only stammer "I got it this summer." And he answered, "That's fine—I'm proud of you!" And gee, for 10 whole minutes I couldn't get my thoughts back to what Dr. Fader was saying.

It's really been quite a day, but I'm disappointed in that I didn't get caught up. 4 new patients, 4–5 to discharge, etc., would have been enough if we didn't have to make so many ward rounds. We made them 3 times—and as usual, each Dr. had different ideas. And as a consequence I didn't get through examining all my new patients. Now perhaps if I were in a stimulating climate, I could have gotten more done.

But I'm at least over the first day and glad of it. Our food is very good, and we already have a favorite waitress who knows I prefer milk to coffee. Stirling Albritton and I are working together in the White Male Ward. Dr. George Bel, director of Medicine and director of the hospital, gave us our pep talk this morning—about how infringements of the rules would be punished by suspension and deprivation of vacation. So I aim to be very good.

Oh, I do miss you so very, very much. I'm hoping to dream of you.

Love,

Alice

OMAHA
Sunday night, July 3
6:50

My darling Alice:

Another chap (Vincent Cedarblade) here is in the same predicament as I am. His fiancée is in Chicago. But that is only 500 miles away, and she is not half as lovely and charming as you are. But I have everything arranged with him. I take his surgery service anytime he goes to see her, and he will take my OB in Sept. And I do hope that you can come.

I got more lonely than ever (if that is possible) last night after I wrote to you, so Cedarblade, a radiology resident named Woodrow Schmela, & I went to a show. Yes, we spent 8 hours salary (25¢) for the show & 3 hours salary for a glass of beer. What extravagance. But the resident is a plutocrat—he gets twice as much pay as we do.

10:45

I had three interns checked out to me tonight, so I have been kept busy writing orders for surgery, seeing patients, etc. Now another OB came in so I suppose it will deliver about 3 a.m.

Our OB resident, Clark McVay, is a swell chap and we are all there for him. Whenever he desires a change in technique, the supt. of nurses does not want to allow it. Charlotte Burgess tries to run the hospital & particularly the OB dept. & still sticks to her methods which she learned in Cook County Hospital some 60 or 70 years ago. And she must not overwork her poor darling nurses.

We had fun with the path resident, Dr. Dave "Bulldog" Drummond. It was his 28th birthday, so we greeted him with the Happy Birthday song as he entered the dining room. Then we presented him with a cake with 6 candles (not that he always acts like a kid).

And again I am looking at the picture of you taken on the boat.

Darling, you are wonderful and I want so much to be near you all of the time. Let us hope that that time is less than a year away.

Mother is worried about you working too hard. And she wonders how your parents are. In every letter she writes about the wonderful time we had down south and what perfect hosts you were. And, of course, she thinks that you are the grandest girl she has ever met.

Again, you have all of my love—

Joe

NEW ORLEANS
Sun. Nite, July 3
8 p.m.

Dearest one—

Today is the biggest red letter day yet. Three letters from you. One I expected yesterday, but two more—well, I've been thrilled over it all day. Dr. Evans—Frances to us—called me to tell me she had been given 2 letters for me, so I came right to my room to read them. Small wonder that I felt so much better than usual this afternoon. I had twice as much reason to be happy.

Your Nu Sig pin has been causing more comment and much staring—from Tulane interns especially. I expect one of them to break down and ask whose pin I have stolen any time now.

Today was an easy day, as I had hoped, and I was able to get off for church. It was the first time I had left the grounds, and I felt as if it were a holiday. I'm really enjoying my work now that I know most of my patients fairly well.

I think I have a much better room than you have from your description. We have hospital beds painted brown, a desk and book-shelf, washstand, and a small—much too small—wardrobe. Our one tiny mirror is about a head too close to the floor and causes us the greatest trouble. But best of all, we have two big windows and it's been cool every night so far—let me knock on wood!

So you read the 13th Chapter of Corinthians. I like it much better with love substituted for charity, as our minister said was done in the latest translations. And doesn't it give one something to live up to!

I had been reading a chapter of the Bible each night during the last school year, but stopped during the summer vacation. What an added joy to know you are reading a chapter every night with me as I begin again.

I think I shall write for my application to Mayo's tonight. And do I have my fingers crossed for good luck! Dr. Jones told me to be sure to write Dr. MacCarty that I was applying. I wonder if it would be too presumptuous to write to Dr. Wilder, too? I hate like the very devil to ask favors of anyone—but I would hate so much more not getting to go to Mayo's. Gosh, 5 of the fellows from last summer there are interning here, and I'm afraid that lessens my chances markedly. Gee, what that fellowship doesn't mean to me!

Good night, dearest, and sweet dreams.

> My love to you,
> Alice

> OMAHA
> Monday the 4th
> 7:00

My dearest:

My morning was full—Surgery, OB & emergencies. In the afternoon I checked out for several hours & played tennis with the OB resident. (The courts are on the hospital grounds.) After four sets of tennis in the blistering heat, then a shower, we had 4 platefuls of orange sherbet for dinner & more iced tea. Well, it cooled us off and it is staying down yet. Perhaps it was not the right thing to do, but it is the Fourth and the sherbet was so good & cold.

And, incidentally, a few interns checked out to me tonight. I have Surgery, Neurology, Ophthalmology, Radiology, Dermatology, Admitting Room, Nose & Throat services on my hands. It is about time for things to start happening. But let's have it. I want work, and I suppose I will see 4-7-8 flashing or short, long, short ringing on my phone.

Incidentally, I took a swell picture of our Dean reading a story to a little girl—won't he like that.

And just now the phone—rats.

9:30

Things really popped. Called to surgery ward & now to admitting room—did I stick my neck out. Gastric carcinoma, indirect inguinal hernia & bursitis on the women. Received a wire that an emergency coming in from Kearney, Neb. More fun & a little work. In the meantime, I'll watch the fireworks from the porch.

> Darling, I love you so much,
> Joe

NEW ORLEANS
Mon. Nite, July 4
8 p.m.

Dearest—

What a Fourth! Dr. Cloyce Huff (from Stanford) signed out on me tonight and Albritton last night. The more the merrier, for then I can perhaps sign out on them sometime in September.

I've been visiting my tuberculosis patients. Poor things, they see an intern so infrequently that they hardly know what to do when I come around. I was called out of bed last night for an old tubercular who was hemorrhaging. Thank goodness it had stopped by the time I got there.

I'll bet you had plenty of work today. It must be quite a service that you are on. I'd really be scared stiff if I had to give even ether anesthesia, much less the other kinds. In fact, ether is the only one I've given—and that only twice.

My dear, how I wish you were one of our "men in white" here, and I could listen for your tick as well as my own (if I could learn it). What great fun it would be!

Until we are really together, I'll always feel you are with me in spirit, too.

All my love for only you—

Alice

OMAHA
Tuesday, July 5
OB staff room, 7:30

My darling:

Talk about deliveries. We have had more than our share. And just as I sat down to eat dinner, another one came. One more patient in labor, so I am waiting to give the anesthetic. The intern did his first episiotomy on the last patient, so it took a lot of ether.

Dr. N.F. Hicken stopped in the middle of an operation this morning and said, "Holoubek, are you still dreaming about that Southern girl?" Why, of course, I was, and I wish that you could have been there in person as well as in spirit.

And, dear, I do hope that you get to take your vacation here in September. I'll get someone to take my OB service. It would be heavenly. Let us hope & pray & it will come true.

Are we having the heat—soon I will drown in my own perspiration. The only time that my room is cool is early in the mornings, but that is usually time to get up.

Dr. Mason, the professor of Tropical Medicine I was telling you about, came to the intern quarters last night & for 2 hours he told stories, such big stories & yet apparently so real & true—and all for the benefit of the OB resident who is not familiar with Mason's ways. But, gee, it was entertaining. Yes, I will remember a few of them to tell you.

My gosh, I wish that patient would deliver.

IN THE QUARTERS

8:55

Dearest:

The patient was getting nowhere fast. I do wish that I could give her ether & take her out of the misery for a few minutes. It will be an episiotomy about 10 or so tonight.

And again I reread your letters—each time with new enjoyment & pleasure. I am so proud to have you wear my pin, dearest.

Tell Dr. Jones that my future plans depend entirely upon you.

I will write for my application at Mayo's tonight. I'll find out all about the personal applications. We must see Mary & Uncle Mac, the Valencia—you must come to Omaha &, above all, Clarkson.

Please don't work too hard.

All my love,

Joe

New Orleans
Tues. Nite, July 5
11:55 p.m.

Dearest—

Just a note this time to tell you how much I love you before I go to bed.

Today has been one full day. I spent all morning on my TB ward. I got to give air to 6 or 8 old patients getting pneumothorax therapy and oil to one. Then Dr. Edgar Hull, my favorite doctor down here, made ward rounds with me. I hear Dr. Hull is soon to have charge of our Medicine service—at least, I hope so. Then I had 2 infusions, a paracentesis, spinal tap, and 10 new patients. I didn't get them quite all worked up, but believe I'll have them by the required 24 hours. I think today must have been a big day for all hospitals.

Being busy all the time does help some but can't take away that longing for you—and those dreams of good times to come. My love is yours. Now goodnight, dearest.

My love,
Alice

Omaha
4:30 Sat afternoon, July 9

My adorable Alice:

It has been very quiet here—only one OB in labor—so we played 3 sets of tennis. I finally got the picture that I promised you—oh, gee, an emergency appendectomy.

6:45

I hope I can finish this letter before something else happens.

One of the residents couldn't believe that you were a physician when I showed him your picture. "They don't make women doctors that nice" was his remark. So I promised that he must meet you and find out for himself how grand you are.

Had another bad night—the OBs come after I get to bed—but I broke a record. It took me 45 seconds from the time I got out of the bed to answer the phone to the time I was in the delivery room. Obviously I did not bother to use the elevator & I combed my hair as I ran through the corridors.

Dearest, it was a year ago last Wednesday that we had our first date—remember that staff meeting? Every moment that I am not near you is time wasted & lost. Darling, my vocabulary is limited when I start to say how much you mean to me, so I will simply say, I love you with my heart & soul.

Joe

Just listening to "Way Down Yonder in New Orleans." What wouldn't I give to be there with you now.

NEW ORLEANS

Tues. Nite, July 12

Darling—

My application blanks from Mayo's came today. Gosh, there's a lot to read over—and a lot that they want that I haven't got. I'm afraid I'm being very presumptuous in applying, but I'm surely going to try. I especially enjoyed the part "Personal applications are enjoyable."

Do I remember that staff meeting—when that fine looking fellow I had been watching in the lab asked me if I wouldn't like to cool off? I surely did want to. But the most peculiar thing to me was how we started talking as if we had known each other all our lives. I remember going in and talking to Mary about you. I remember telling her especially about what fine ideals and ideas you had—that started me off. Poor Mary, she had to listen to me rave, but I know she enjoyed it too—'specially after she had met you and could agree with me. And she had quite a job consoling me that night after you came to tell me good-bye.

Ah, we have lots to be thankful for even if there are those awful 1,103 miles. Thank goodness for your letters—and the feeling of your caring and being with me always. It means so much to me.

My love,

Alice

NEW ORLEANS

Wed. Nite, July 13

My dearest one—

Your picture gets better each time I look at it—which is very often,
I assure you. My, but you were all dressed up—and well you deserve
to be. Every time I think of you, an M.D. at the age of 22, I'm
amazed all over again. Gee, I'm so proud of you—and how I do love
you. I'm going to read over the chapter in Corinthians again and
see if I have the right to say I love you. And you, spending 8 hours
salary at a show. If you think that is extravagant, what do you think
about us? We spend 23 hours salary when we go. Oh, my, how will I
ever get rich at this rate?

I feel like a slacker today. I quit working at 8:00 this p.m. And
the nurses tell us that we have been coming to the ward too early
in the morning, that things aren't ready for us until 9 o'clock, so I
think I'm going to start getting up later. Dr. Fader has been kidding
me because I don't sit down to give infusions, feel for spleens, take
blood pressure, etc. He says he's trying to teach me—and I'm slowly
learning to do it, when I have plenty of time.

Hooray! Kay Kyser tonight. Remember? We heard that show
together on our first night in Alexandria. Oh, dear, what sweet
memories we do have—and how I'm hoping to collect some more
sweet ones in September. Imagine, seeing your hospital, Clarkson,
your home, Rochester—and best of all, you.

All my love,

Alice

OMAHA
Thursday, July 14
8:05

My darling:

Bing Crosby & Bob Burns—I do hope that you are listening. And perhaps they will play "You Leave Me Breathless." But any love song reminds me of you.

And on my desk I have the picture folder Romantic New Orleans. How true. Any place with you would be romantic. But that Louisiana moon with you beside me—who could ask for anything more? Yes, I am so very jealous of the moon as I look at it out of my window at night—it can look down upon you.

Had another OB last night. They always come at the time when it is coolest to sleep. Yes, the anesthetist is usually as much asleep as the patient.

Had a full a.m. Even got in on orthopedic clinic & got to set a dislocated shoulder. Aw, rats—there is a call from the admitting room. Until later—

All my love,
Joe

10:30

Dearest:

A full evening's work. An outpatient in admitting room. Diagnosis is measles. I hope I'm right but it is typical. Then an OB came in—will deliver sometime tonight. A patient gone hysterical on surgery with amytal and other things to keep me going. Yes, I'm up to my usual standard—4 fellows checked out to me tonight.

I am rather glad that I have this service first. I can learn OB & surgery technique from observation, and I have been checked in on practically every service, so I should know the ropes by the time that I get on them.

I may take a few hours off & go home in a few weeks. But we will go for more than a few hours when you come down.

Darling, if I could be with you from this moment on to the end of time, it would not be long enough.

I love you,
Joe

New Orleans
Thurs. Nite, July 14

Dearest—

What a day! Ward rounds all morning, Salvarsan clinic for syphilitics from 12:30 to 2:30—and 5 new patients and one readout to work up. But I'm quite elated. I did my first spinal taps today—and was I surprised to see the fluid drip out! It was so much easier than I expected, but I didn't feel that impulse you are supposed to when you enter the spinal canal. We were supposed to do one on one of my patients, a chronic alcoholic, but he said he had seen too many done and that he was sure it would kill him, and he deserted rather than have one.

I have two tubercular patients who will probably expire tonight so I'm expecting some calls. Say, it sounds to me as if you are being kept pretty busy. Remember, please don't work too hard!

You give me a new happy thought in saying you hope you can spend our two weeks vacation together. That would be heavenly. I can't permit myself to think too much about our September week, for I get so anxious for it to come that I can't bear the thought of waiting so long.

Goodnight, my dear. I'll soon be with you in my dreams.

All my love,
Alice

OMAHA
Friday night, July 15
10:00

My adorable Alice:

Another day away from you—it seems so empty. Many things have been accomplished, but without you at my side it seems so useless. My great inspiration is that I am doing it for you and someday we can work together.

Received a very interesting letter from A.C. He enjoys work very much. He says that Uncle Mac is a great person, an inspirational teacher, as well as a very radical individual. Here is what he wrote: "He thought it was great stuff when I said that you had been down to see Alice Baker. He remembered both of you. He said, 'Other things besides pathology are being promoted in this lab.'"

I am anxiously awaiting the time when you and I will walk together to see him. Won't I be so very proud.

A.C. is having Drs. H.K. Gray & Charles Mayo help him with his thesis, but he didn't tell me what he was writing about.

And A.C. had quite a time with Dr. Adson. It seems that Adson tied off the internal carotid & asked one of the path regular Fellows about the collateral circulation & he didn't know, so he pointed to A.C., who described the Circle of Willis arteries. Adson was astounded. When he found out A.C. was from Nebraska, he spent a lot of time telling the gallery of the fine anatomy course here. Gee, I would have liked to have seen that—with fellows from Harvard & Northwestern standing & watching. Did Dean Poynter like that when I told him! He beamed from ear to ear. And I am so proud of A.C. I am surely lucky that he did not ask me that question last year or he might have received a different impression of Nebraska anatomy.

As I sit here with my application to Mayo's beside me, I dream that we will be there together. Dearest, what & when are you going to apply for? I plan to apply for internal medicine. It is true that I have not had all of my clinical work yet & am not certain of the specialty, but I favor medicine now. Darling, we could work together in any line—and I hope & pray that we will both get in next year.

I also read the part about "personal interviews with applicants are desirable." I can just see us walking in to see Dr. Wilder. I bet he would recall us from the Thursday afternoon clinics at Curie Hospital & the Wednesday ward rounds at St. Marys. And wouldn't Uncle Mac's eyes pop.

You must meet Dr. Poynter. I sat in his office for 1 hour today & he expounded on everything from Mayo's, internships, hospitals, modern medicine, and finally exploded on medical education of the laymen by newspaper columns, magazines & movies. What a character he is.

I feel that I left part of myself down there with you, & I am so sorry that I cannot be there all of the time.

> A goodnight kiss & my love,
> Joe

Omaha
Sunday, July 17
2:00

My darling:

Drummond took a beating last night. He left this morning for 2 weeks in Reserve Officer's camp at Ft. Crook, 20 miles south of here, so he went out to celebrate last night. So we fixed up his room, stuffed his suit & shirt, fixed shoes & boots, put on an officer's cap, Sam Browne belt, brush for a sword, and fixed a broom for the horse. On the door was written "Lt. 'Buck' Drummond rides again and again, 25¢ per person." Then we filled the remaining space & bed with laundry boxes stacked to the ceiling. What a picture—yes, I took some. Well, "Buck" came in early this morning & stormed into every room switching on lights, etc., looking for an empty bed. He took it as a joke, but I fear he will bring the entire regiment back with him next week.

We do have a lot of fun here but, darling, it is nothing considering the good times that I am missing with you. It would be heavenly if I could hold you in my arms once more and receive a kiss from you. This is our lot for one more year to be separated, but let us hope that we can see each other for two perfect weeks during that time. And after that, darling, arm in arm always.

I wish we could go to Gluck's Restaurant for a soft shell crab dinner—later for a West Indian daiquiri & then for some shrimp & beer.

My love,
Joe

NEW ORLEANS

Tues. evening, July 19

Dearest one—

I have a most interesting case now. He came in in a state of restlessness and slight irrationality (is there such a word?). Anyway, I soon decided it was useless to try to get a history, and then I discovered his blood pressure was 210/110. So with the help of the admitting room diagnosis, I diagnosed my first case of hypertensive encephalopathy. Later he had a convulsion, and we've really been working on him. The diagnosis may be changed to uremia, however, because he has elevated albumen, many casts and a few red blood cells in his urine. At any rate, it is a very interesting case.

Dot just came in. She's on emergency duty tonight and has really been working. She's been watching the reports on the chest X-rays of the interns and says they've found 2 active TB cases and 6 or 8 whom they are calling inactive or latent. Gee, that's surely something I have to be thankful for—a negative one.

I'm still enjoying the pneumothorax work at Dibert. Dr. Hull tickles me. One time he calls me Dr. Baker and the next Alice or Miss Alice. I hope he will send a recommendation to Mayo's for me, for I would value his more than anyone else's.

Goodnight, my dear, and all my love.

Alice

Omaha
Wed., July 20
6:35

Dearest Alice:

What a day—I never had my number flashed so many times. Surgery from 7:45 to 2 p.m. and then finally lunch. And now another anesthetic scheduled for 7 p.m. Gee, it is fun, but the only thing that I don't like about is that I only got to read your letter three times during the day.

Did I have a scare today. An appendectomy, heavily narcotized, and I gave cyclopropane. Suddenly he quit breathing and for five minutes—which seemed like five years—I gave CO_2 & O_2 and artificial respiration. And what a relief when I saw that first gasp, and then another, and finally, regular respirations. Hot dog, what an experience. I'd rather not repeat it every day.

Twenty days of internship gone—that much closer to next summer and what it holds in store for us. Darling, we must have faith that the dreams will come true.

Tommy Dorsey is signing off, which means it is 7 p.m. and time to go to surgery or my telephone will ring off the wall.

My love,
Joe

NEW ORLEANS
Wed. Night, July 20

Dearest Joe—

We had good news today. We hear that Dr. Hull is going to be our visiting man from now on. I'm so glad. We'll probably find ourselves working twice as hard and not minding half as much.

Our resident pulled one on me today. It's the custom in the dining hall to give the gong to any intern who stops to speak to a resident or who comes in dressed in civilian clothes or does anything else unusual. So as I walked in tonight all unsuspectingly, Dr. Clarence Bishop called me to his table. I thought of it as I got halfway there and just started to say, "If you cause me to get the gong"— when he started it himself. Gee, was I embarrassed! Just wait, I'll get him back some way.

I lost another TB patient today and am expecting another at any minute. The fellow who had a marked hemoptysis started coughing up blood again tonight. He had just told me that tomorrow is his birthday. I hope he lives to celebrate one more.

Have you heard of the new antigen used for a skin test for tuberculosis which doesn't contain the TB organism? I hear it's supposed to be as sensitive as tuberculosis without the chance of flaring up an infection. It sounds good and I hope to get the chance to try it.

It seems ages since I've told you that I love you and since I've heard it from you—but here's hoping it won't be much longer, dear.

All my love—
Alice

NEW ORLEANS
Thurs. Night, July 21

Dearest one—

I told Henry Jernigan, one of our Tulane friends, my plans for
September tonight and does he envy me! He asked about you and
said he wanted me to do a lot of talking for him while I was in
Rochester. It seems he had a very enjoyable time in Rochester also.
Gosh, I do so hope everything comes out alright. I'm getting mighty
scared that I won't get that fellowship. I was talking to our intern
from Stanford who has a cousin and a friend up there. He wants to
go there too but says it is so difficult for someone to get in after just
one year's internship that he isn't even going to try until he has at
least one more year in a hospital. I can't see why you should have
any difficulty in getting in, especially with that wonderful thesis to
your credit, but I can't see much chance for myself. However, I'm
still hoping.

Darling, I'll be seeing you soon in my dreams. Remember me to
your folks—and all my love to you.

Alice

OMAHA
Sat. night, July 23
9:30

Sweetheart:

Cedarblade & I just came up from the wards and then, since both of us are so lonely, we couldn't get started writing our letters soon enough. He is going to Chicago in one or two weeks, lucky chap. If I only had wings, darling, I'd be at your side tonight.

Another Saturday night and, as usual, I have 5 or 6 services on my hands, so my short, long, short will be keeping me awake tonight, for there is no hour that the interns must be in. Most of the married ones check out for the night.

Had an OB case go into shock on the table. Pulse 140, blood pressure 90/50. But CO_2 + O_2, intravenous glucose, etc., pulled her out—and was McVay glad to see the nurses have things ready.

I am so glad that Dr. Hull treats you so nicely. There is nothing better than having the visiting man help you and advise you as much as possible.

The 13th Chapter of Corinthians has proven quite a consolation to me, and soon I will know it by heart. When it says that "Love (charity) beareth all things, believeth all things, hopeth all things, endureth all things and never falleth away"—darling, ours must be that way.

You have my heart.

Joe

NEW ORLEANS
Sat. Night, July 23

My dearest one—

How I love to write that! And how I love to see your greetings on
my letters—but darling, you make me happiest yet when you tell
me that you love me. Dearest, we are having a bumpy road as far as
being apart so much goes, but I know that in having your love I am
the most fortunate person on this universe.

I really had decided that there was no one whom I could find
who would live up to my yardstick. I've always known that I could
never truly care for anyone whom I couldn't respect—and there
were so many things I wanted my one to have—and I truly thought
I was expecting too much. But, darling, knowing you I realize that
I did not ask for too much. In you I have found more than anyone
could ever desire. Just knowing you has been the finest thing in my
life. Such inane raving—and you, poor dear, can't defend yourself.
Let me try to get back to earth again.

A sad thing happened on the ward today. A patient, 55 years of
age, who had been very ill with a kidney infection, was scheduled
to go home today. He didn't want to leave the hospital, but I'm sure
you've seen enough of Charity to understand that we can't keep
patients after we have gotten them afebrile and in a condition that
they can be cared for at home. Well, they put him in a rolling chair,
and he suddenly had a stroke. He is still unconscious and I've just
been talking to his son. It was quite pitiful.

I still fear old age more than anything else. Helplessness in one
who has led a fine life is the most pitiful thing I can think of. The
inimitableness of life—ah, it's too much for me. And I'm thankful
for my scenes of complete happiness which are being woven in my
life by knowing you.

Thanks again, dear, for being whom and what you are—and for
caring about me.

Love,
Alice

OMAHA
Mon. night, July 25
8:25

My darling:

Another long dreary day away from you. How dreadfully long they seem. And only a few enjoyable moments—those when I read my letter from you. But I did have a very pleasant dream this p.m. I had a few moments to spare and fell asleep for a few minutes. In that time I lived years and years with you. It was wonderful.

About Rochester—it is so very true that 1-year fellows are rarely accepted—but it has been done, so why can't we? But if we fail, I have decided on a residency at Charity—and that may be harder for me to crack than Mayo's. I could not stand another year away from you. Or would you want to take advanced work elsewhere? However, we are going to get to Mayo's next year, and the trip there in September will get us in. Further, it will bring us together for 4 or 5 heavenly days.

Heard from A.C. again. Uncle Mac was to have a lawn party for the group last Saturday but it was postponed due to the death of Mrs. David Berkman (Drs. Wm. & Chas. Mayo's sister). He also rode down the elevator with Mrs. Roosevelt and he says, "She's just a well dentaled babe."

My heart to you,
Joe

New Orleans
Mon. Night, July 25

Dearest one—

We had a meeting today at which the interns and residents in LSU Med were given a new set of rules—in addition to those for all interns. Aside from the fact that we practically have to have our signature witnessed by a resident each time we want to write our name, they are very nice.

Did I have fun today. Dr. Howles, our chief of dermatology—a huge blond fellow who has been very nice to me—had been looking at our skin patients with me when he suddenly said, "Say, isn't that a NΣN pin?" I said it was. "Who is it?" I told him very proudly. "What, not one of our boys?" "No, sir." "Well, is he nice—nice enough for you?" "Oh, yes," I beamed. Then he turned around to me and yelled, "Congratulations!" I'm sure everyone in the ward heard him, but I was beaming so I forgot to be embarrassed.

Nice enough for me? Darling, you're too darned nice for me, but I can love you even so—and do love you and hope to dream of you tonight.

With all my heart,
Alice

Omaha
Tue. Night, July 26

My darling:

Had an awfully bad night and day. As I completed your letter last evening, an acute appendix came in, followed by some minor surgery, and then another acute appendix. I finally got to bed at 1:30 only to be awakened at 4 a.m. for an OB. About the time I got through with the last anesthetic I felt like I could have an appendectomy performed on me without any anesthetic whatsoever. Isn't it odd that things come in waves like that & undoubtedly nothing will happen tonight & I'll have all night to dream of you.

Took a couple of hours off this p.m. and accomplished an awful lot. First, I had to appear before the examining board before I receive my commission in ROTC, and to my surprise, the board consisted of Col. Lynn Hall & Col. Floyd Nelson, both Nu Sigs and very good friends of mine. I took them hunting pheasants to Clarkson for three years. After an interchange of greetings, Col. Hall said, "No questions. It's up to you, Col. Nelson." And he replied, "I have none." So you see, it was simple. But I had to promise to take them to Clarkson this fall & that mother would have some kolaches for them.

Finally to see Dr. George Pratt, one of our Medical Chiefs, about Mayo's. "What do you want to go there for—you have 1 chance in a thousand" was his first remark.

But after I had told him of my connections & last summer there, he advised applying and said he would recommend me. Darling, we will have Drs. MacCarty, Wilder, Adson, Hench, Allen & more pulling for us. Gee, we must get in. But we must not be too hopeful.

I wish they would complete remodeling our dining room here. We are eating in very crowded quarters now and have breakfasts with the nurses to boot. The interns & residents & staff eat together. But any intern gets the razz if he stops to talk to a nurse here in the dining room.

Heard from Mother today. Apparently the grasshoppers are bad at home, but last night's rain probably broke the drought.

Darling, soon I will gaze holes through the pictures of you that I have in my room. And may I have one of your application photos? Mine are not taken yet.

> Sweetheart—I adore you,
> Joe

NEW ORLEANS
Thurs. nite, July 28

Dearest one—

What a night. Frances invited us to her home for dinner—and did
we have a delicious feast. Fried chicken, avocado salad, potatoes,
corn, lima beans, and a huge dish of ice cream. My, we did enjoy it,
especially after this hospital fare. Then we went riding. We drove
out to Pontchartrain Beach park, rode the "Bug," ate popcorn, drank
beer—and talked about you.

I am so very pleased that you sent me those pictures. They are
marvelous. Your sister looks so much like your mother. I'm so anxious to know her. And yours—it is so good of you it almost hurts
when I look at it, for it makes me miss you so much I can hardly
stand it. I really don't see how I can leave it in my room all day while
I'm working. I'll just have to be running up all the time to look at it.

I read the 13th chapter of Corinthians to Dot last night—I just
had to share it with someone—and we both enjoyed it. To know
that you are reading it too makes it very precious to me.

Darling, again, words can't express how I am looking forward to
seeing you and how deeply I miss you now. And oh, how very much
I love you.

Alice

OMAHA
Fri. night, July 29
9:15

My adorable darling:

I had a swell time after dinner tonight. It rained—a steady, heavy rain like we had down in N.O. I went walking and got royally soaked, but it was a lot of fun. I only wished that you would be here. It would be wonderful, doing the things that we both enjoy.

One more day on anesthesia—and another 7:30 a.m. case. Dr. William L. Shearer decided to come earlier today so I missed breakfast, & surgery kept me there until 2 p.m. Isn't it funny how one forgets about food or sleep when he is doing things that he enjoys? And even though Dr. Shearer bawls out everyone in the room and always demands the Shearer needle & needle holder, raves about the Shearer cast, & about Dr. Shearer—nevertheless, his surgery is superb and he is a master at cleft palate & harelips.

Call from admitting room—OB in.

11:25

A placenta previa—confirmed by X-ray. The hemorrhage has stopped, donors are being typed—but I fear that I may have to get up for a caesarean sometime tonight.

Now to Jan Garber with "Naturally Dreams Come True." Darling, my dreams of September are endless. Until I hold you tightly (so tightly) in my arms—

I love you,
Joe

ОМАНА
Sat. night, July 30

My darling:

Just got ready to take Ernie Cerv & his fiancée to a show. He is a
senior in medicine & she a junior. Yes, I have been telling her about
you & LSU and you and AEI and you & N.O. Yes, everything about
you, but I fear that my description is not half nice enough.

Planned to go home tomorrow but received a note from Mother
saying that she and father are coming over tomorrow. Now if you
would be here the day would be complete. I cannot wait until we'll
be together, my dearest.

Love,
Joe

ОМАНА
Sunday, July 31
5:55

My darling:

Father and Mother just went home in Nola—we had a wonderful
time. They came at 11 a.m. We had a picnic lunch with fried chicken,
kolaches & cherry pie. And, of course, we had Evangeline sauce.
Darling, we missed you and your parents so much. Later we visited
the parks & airport and the hospital. Needless to say, the main topic
of discussion was what a perfect time we had at your home with your
lovely parents & you. Mother is worried that you are working too
hard—and I agree with her. Please take things easy, dear.

Now I am more lonely than ever—gee, I need you, darling. But,
in September it will be grand.

Call from receiving room—

11:30

Dearest:

What a night. Imagine my surprise when I came down to the emergency room & saw my father & mother there cut up & bruised. Some crazy darn drunk hit them while they were going along about 40 in the outermost lane. Father had bruised knees & a hurt back, while Mother had a laceration on the scalp, lip & knee. They were not unconscious. Pulse & respiration were OK, but needless to say they were severely shaken up. Got them fixed up, and with the help of a little sedation, they should rest until morning.

Now a call from OB.

OB Ward

Darling:

Waiting for a delivery—primipara, 5 fingers dilated.

Where was I? Oh, I suppose in the middle of the accident. Well, we have a lawyer & plan to have a hearing tomorrow. We have insurance but the drunk doesn't. So what—probably a judgement, but it means nothing.

Yes, Nola has a few scratches—in fact, several hundred dollars worth—but by the time you see her she will be the same sweet, obedient Nola.

But gee, we are so very lucky that it was not any worse. Thank God. At times like this we must realize that we are being protected by the Maker. When I think how bad it could have been—gee, we are lucky.

I hope these two OBs pop off fast so that I could get some sleep.

Darling, I am counting the days until you will be here.

Love,

Joe

Omaha
10:30 Mon. night, Aug.1

My dearest:

It is surprising how a busy evening on admitting room followed by about 8 Oto-Rhino-Laryngology consultations enable an individual to forget how blue he should be. I like my nose & throat service but have not had the opportunity to do much yet. Should get to do a lot of surgery if I get the right staff man.

I do hope that I never have to spend another night & day like yesterday & today. Of course, the folks felt worse today than yesterday and had more pains. Mother will have a scar on her scalp and one on the knee to remind her of the day. Dad's knees are a bit stiff. What they need now is a good rest at home for several days. Yes, they took Nellie home at 4 p.m. today.

Went out to the scene of the accident today & took pictures of the area. Then followed the preliminary hearing. We have a clear-cut case with sufficient witnesses, but the defendant has no insurance or money. Gosh, after looking at that car again, I don't see how they got out alive. The only thing left is the seat. And thanks to Dad's strong arms, the car stayed on the road even though he bent the steering wheel doing it. Yes, it's quite a loss. Nola seemed so much a part of us—why, she was one of the family. And now—well, she saved Mother and Dad's lives with her sturdy construction and shatterproof glass. What nobler deed could she have done? I'll have the appraiser look at her tomorrow.

Again I thank God because we were so fortunate.

There, I did not mean to bore you with all of my troubles—but, as you may notice, they are a burden now.

How welcome your letters were today—Darling, new inspiration & hope coming from you. And now I keep my chin up and no one knows that anything happened. But I wish that I could be near my folks and cheer them up tonight.

The days are coming closer and closer and soon you will be in my arms again.

Joe

New Orleans
Wednesday, Aug. 3

My dearest one—

I was so sorry to hear of your folks' accident. Do let me know how they are getting along—I surely hope nothing serious results. It must have been a terrible shock to find them in the emergency room. I too am so thankful that it was no worse than it was. It is my prayer that you and yours be continually watched after by our Lord—you are certainly deserving.

I have a most interesting case of mycosis fungoides. The skin lesions are most bizarre appearing and the patient is in pretty bad shape. He has a lesion on his left tonsil, in his nose, and we think perhaps the areas of infiltration in his lungs are due to the same process. He is suffering now from severe asthmatic attacks. As soon as we can get an ENT man to examine him, we hope to determine if there is some tracheo-bronchial obstruction causing the asthma.

As I told Bernes, I'm more than ready for September to come. She and Dot both asked me to tell you how sorry they were to hear about your parents. I hope to hear from you tomorrow that they are feeling alright again. They could have no better care than their son's.

Goodnight, my love,
Alice

NEW ORLEANS
Fri. nite, Aug. 5

Dearest—

I was delighted to hear that your parents were able to go home today. They certainly are courageous to start right out again in Nellie. I surely hope their injuries aren't very painful. I can't understand how they were that fortunate after your description of the accident. But how thankful I am. Gee, your folks seem very close to me now and I do think so much of them.

We had stuffed crabs for dinner. Guess whom that reminded me of? But they weren't nearly so good as those of New Iberia. Oh, do you suppose we can ever relive those days—at least we can in our dreams.

I was very disappointed today. The patient with mycosis fungoides died this noon, and his family wouldn't let me have an autopsy—so I'll never know if he had tuberculosis of the lung, or a lesion of the mycosis fungoides variety.

I do hate to beg for autopsies for I know I wouldn't want to give permission for an autopsy on anyone I cared for, even though I wouldn't mind one on myself. In fact, I'm still trying to figure out a way to see my own autopsy. Homer Dupuy, our crack impersonator, won the prize for securing the most autopsies last month—6 with 7 deaths. He could sell cracked ice to an Eskimo and enjoy doing it. Wish I had more of that ability.

I hope your folks are better. Remember me to them.

All my love,
Alice

NEW ORLEANS

Wed. Nite, Aug. 10

My dearest—

There is nothing I enjoy more than coming in from the ward tired and finding a letter from you. I read it over and over and have a pleasurable time dreaming of you. Then I feel as if I could go out and work harder than ever.

Dr. Huff had a mishap today. As he was giving air to one of his TB patients, he suddenly keeled over himself. When he came around he started vomiting and has kept it up all day. I don't like those symptoms, do you? He is looking better tonight and wants to come back to work tomorrow, but I doubt if they let him. Albritton and I are dividing his work—of which there hasn't been much as yet, thank goodness.

And I've done 16 of my 18 TB patients' sputum. Thank goodness I'll soon be through with those—for a month, at any rate.

Mother says Ray may get transferred from New York to the Veterans Hospital in Chillicothe, Ohio. If so, she will probably go there to help him make the move. I hope Marie will be able to stand it all right. At least they will be a little closer to home.

Our ward is overflowing again. I guess I'll have several patients to discharge tomorrow. I really wish we could keep some of them longer and see how they get along, but we have to send them out as soon as it is possible. It is funny how hard it is to get some of them home. One boy has been discharged for about three weeks and hasn't gone yet. Poor fellow, he has congenital polycystic lung with multiple abscesses—and his folks have no money to take care of him. Gee, won't it be great if the recession ever lets up.

How I would enjoy a good talk with you—or just to look at you. And until I can, I'll be dreaming of it.

Love,

Alice

OMAHA
Thu. Night, Aug. 11
12:00 midnight

My dearest:

Got another acute abdomen in tonight, and it had better be a perforated ulcer. Called a staff man & he should be out about 12:30. I am going to see that operation if it takes till morning. I should get a book on "acute abdomen." When I wrote my senior comprehensive examination on it, it all seemed so easy. But when one of these cases comes in on an ambulance, it seems that all of the little I learned leaves me. Yes, my errors on acute tummies are frequent.

Had a lot of fun doing an autopsy with Drummond tonight. Gee, I learned more anatomy, & actually felt the epiploic foramen & other things that I heard about in anatomy years ago. And it was fun with the brain. I learned a lot of neurology—but I still cannot see how Dr. Adson can tell the 7th from the 9th cranial nerves or others. I also got permission to assist on any other autopsies—more fun.

Gee, 200 admissions in one day would fill up our institution. We admit all day & night but on Tuesday & Friday p.m., I have ORL surgery, so the intern on anesthetic takes over the emergencies & the admissions wait. At times like that I go through them in a hurry.

The fellows don't mind my missed diagnoses. They say "Well, he was dreaming of the South & his girl again."

I love you,
Joe

OMAHA
Sunday night, Aug.14
8:45

My darling:

I went home today. Left at 7 a.m., arrived at 10, took the bus back from Schuyler at 6 p.m.

Father and Mother are just getting over their severe shaking up. They lost a lot of weight and are just regaining their appetites. Mother still limps. Gee, I do hope that she comes out of it soon. Undoubtedly the nervous shock was more than I had anticipated.

Father does not talk much as a rule, but he surely let out quite a lecture today on the hazard of drunken drivers and the inadequacy of our highway patrol. "Why, they don't drive like that in Louisiana. Their police force is more effective."

Dennis's hair is turning blond from red—too bad. He should be able to walk by the time that you come in September.

The corn was "firing"—our term meaning burned by the hot wind. I do hope that the rain that we had tonight will cool things off. Again I like La. since it rains there every day.

Nola is no more. It broke my heart to part with her, but she lived a noble life. Her spirit will live on. Memories of Nola & you will live forever.

Now, Nola's place is taken by a 1938 commander State Sedan. She is wonderful—free wheeling, overdrive and all, including our radio. It's a thrill to drive her. I took her home. The folks will get more use of her. But we will use her in September. Build up our dreams and lives and future around her.

Love,

Joe

NEW ORLEANS
Mon. Nite, Aug. 15

Dearest one—

Well, I've had one guess come out right. A patient came in because of an attack of vomiting, with a history of such attacks of similar character for 3½ years. When I saw the fixed and unequal pupils, my diagnosis of syphilis was made—and in spite of negative Wasserman's test and presence of knee-jerk reflexes, I stuck to it, for I had no idea what else it could possibly be. So today I got his old chart and he had had a strongly positive Wasserman—blood and spinal fluid—in 1935, with a similar attack and had even been given malaria to induce fever. Now at least I've seen what gastric crises can look like.

Frances phoned me this afternoon and insisted (you can imagine how much she had to insist) that I come to her home for dinner tonight, and gee, did I enjoy it! Good old fried chicken—yum, yum. I just hope I didn't make too much of a pig of myself. Then we went to the Country Club to swim. I surely feel my lack of exercise, for a couple of hundred yards and I was out of breath. I surely enjoyed it, though, and thanks to Frances' membership there, we hope to do it often.

Of course, we had to have some beer, too. It seems that Frances gets a commission or something on Regal beer. At any rate, we did our part.

Dearest, I miss you more and more, and how I am looking forward to our week together. My, I can hardly wait. Will you promise not to get tired of hearing me say I love you?

Alice

OMAHA
Fri. night, Aug. 19
11:05

My darling:

That pediatrics ward appears more like a mad house. I have a few ORL patients there. But I do enjoy the work with children.

We had a couple of emergency ORL cases (bronchoscopy & mastoidectomy) added to our schedule this p.m., so we had a very full operative schedule. I still cannot see how or when they know when they are near the dura mater or trans sinus or facial nerve in some of those radical mastoidectomies.

Had an interesting brain case come in. Headache for several months with increased drowsiness. A ventricular puncture decompression revealing a malignant brain tumor done this p.m. Dr. J.J. Keegan did the work. I was rather surprised to see him come out at 2 a.m. He is a classmate of Dr. Adson and does good work. He keeps a poker face & never says anything. In fact, all during the procedure he never tells much what he finds.

Got my reply from Mayo's this p.m. Gee, the applications will not be considered until in April—my gosh, that is late. After that it will be pretty late to get something else. Perhaps I could get into the army at Fort Snelling in St. Paul so that I could be near you. But, we must have faith, & in April we will both receive the welcome news, I hope, I pray.

Gee, my summer vacation seems so much like a dream, Alexandria & New Orleans a sort of dream world. But, dearest, you are real and so must everything else connected with you be. It is so wonderful. And our dreams for the future.

From the bottom of my heart, I adore you.

Joe

OMAHA
12:20 Sunday night, Aug. 21

My darling:

Almost got locked in the ice box while I was searching for some ice cream, but the cook was kind enough to rescue me. I got the ice cream, but it turned out to be sherbet.

Had a dullish day but during the evening we had several accident cases. Had a girl with a cut arm. I'd have given a lot to have been allowed to fix it, but they wanted a private M.D. so she was taken to another hospital. Darn it.

I also fixed up a sprained wrist for the Barnes & Sells-Floto circus people, so the fellow scattered free tickets to tonight's show around the admitting room. And believe me, we disappeared in a hurry & went to the circus. The hospital lost most of the interns.

My gosh, what a show—the largest I have ever seen. There were dozens of good acts. However, I did wonder how hard it would be to do an esophageal dilatation on the giraffe.

It does seem odd, but I can stand in surgery & watch Dr. Adson or Keegan do a brain tumor and know that a slip of the retractor would mean death to the patient & I get no thrill out of it, but when I watch some of the nutty performers do some balancing acts with nothing but hard ground 75 feet below, I get a swell case of apnea. Gee, I could find a much safer place to make a living than the circus. But then we do surgery or autopsies on virulent strep cases with only a rubber glove & a thin layer of epithelium between us & the infectious organism. No, we are not safe either—but I prefer this.

Darling, you certainly have influenced every moment of my life. Why, even a circus, the thing that I always enjoyed, is flat and empty without you there with me. Even a glass of beer tastes sour when I drink it without you. I adore you and am counting the days until I will hold you in my arms. And please don't work too hard.

My love,

Joe

OMAHA
Mon. night, Aug. 22
11:45

My darling:

What a day. Two new ORL patients, in addition to some consultations. More fun.

A penny ante poker game has been going on. How odd. Last year no one played for less than a nickel or a dime, but now it is pennies. One fellow "lost his shirt"—20¢.

Drummond's room looked a mess the other night. He announced his engagement, so we conveniently sprinkled rice all over everything.

Later McVay's wife came to town from St. Louis, and the next a.m. Mac found all of his furniture out in the corridor. Nothing is safe with this gang. It is all in fun. But one thing that they don't dare bother, & that is your picture. I would lose my temper if they'd take that.

Please forgive me if I cut this short, darling, but I was up with admitting room a lot of last night & this morning, and we have two more cases due tonight.

My dear, it seems so very, very long since I have held your hand—oh, I adore you.

My love,
Joe

NEW ORLEANS
Tues. Nite, Aug. 23

My dearest—

Ah, another bit of teasing from the boys. They tell me I had better be careful about having my letters sent to the intern quarters, especially those from Omaha, Neb., as it is too tempting to read them. Ha—they had just better let me catch them reading your letters. But anything to tease me about.

I saw a case today of originally minimal tuberculosis who had been kept in bed at Dibert for one year. She had been doing so well that she was told she could go home after one more X-ray. But that last plate showed more extensive infiltration and several small cavities. Gosh, what a disease! Thank goodness I'll soon be off that service—which certainly isn't spoken as a true physician.

Oh, darling, tomorrow I request my vacation—and what does that mean to me?—a week of heaven on earth. Don't work too hard helping everyone else, darling, and remember, I love you.

Alice

NEW ORLEANS
Thurs a.m., Aug. 25

My dearest—

Please forgive the short note this is going to be for it is 1:30 a.m. Now, don't feel sorry for me, I haven't been working. My brother Ray drove down to see me—quite a nice surprise—and luckily I could check out. We left about 2 p.m. and just got in. As you know, he interned at Hotel Dieu and had to visit all his friends, from undertakers thru dentists, doctors, etc. The only thing which bothered me was that everywhere we went, they insisted we have something to drink—and Ray egged me on, too. However, I'm still here, none the worse for it, I hope—and probably the better, for it ended up with me again telling myself that I really do not care for the stuff and will certainly not drink, at least not unless the social occasion demands it, which apparently happens more often in New Orleans than elsewhere. Anyway, I don't like it and wish Ray didn't like it quite so much.

Gee, I've wasted all this time talking about that and I've got to get to bed, for tomorrow is a busy day. This, thank goodness, doesn't take much room to say—"I love you." So I can say it over and over again.

Darling, all enjoyments are so incomplete without you, and how complete every moment is with you.

Goodnight, dearest,
Alice

Omaha
Thu. Night, Aug. 25

My sweetheart:

Gee, what a session—just got the last intern out of my room. And the air is still thick with Drummond's stories of Montana, Schmela & last year's interns. Lucky McVay wasn't in or we would have heard about St. Louis again. They are a grand bunch of fellows.

I can hear chips flying in the poker game. Stakes are high—nickel limit.

I had been crying $45 tears the past 2 days because I had lost my ophthalmoscope. I asked everyone in the hospital from the janitors up to the physicians. And tonight Drummond asked if I had use for my 'scope. Yes, a playful chap—just wondering how soon I'd need it after he found it 2 days ago. Now he comes in complaining of finding his books all over the bed—now who would possibly do such a thing?

Received a request for $1 to renew my Neb. medical license. My gosh, I just got through paying $25 for it & now they want more.

Soon we will be in Rochester together—perhaps at the Valencia. What a place to relive happy moments. How about a reunion for the entire group of 1937? Perhaps Mary Giffin will be home yet. Uncle Mac should be back from his vacation by then.

I am so anxious to have everyone here meet you, Dearest. Until then I will keep telling them about you.

I love you,

Joe

New Orleans

Thursday, Aug. 25

My darling—

I have just ruined about six sheets of paper trying to write a satisfactory request for our personal application. I do so want it to be right—and everything to come out right.

Oh, I got so lonesome once for you tonight that I could hardly stand it. Dr. Bishop's girlfriend called him up, and I couldn't help hearing—I assure you I wasn't eavesdropping—but gosh, for a moment I wanted to hear your voice so badly that I was very glad I could bend my head over my chart so no one could see me. That faraway look would have been too evident to anyone.

Today I also requested my week's vacation. I understand I'm ahead of anyone else asking for that time, so I should have no trouble.

Ray said, "Well, what about the boyfriend?" So I told him—at great length and frequent intervals. He wishes us the best of luck.

Dr. Hull told me yesterday that he had gotten a letter from Mayo's asking for a recommendation. And LSU's Dean Ophelia (Stone) Stone—have I told you about her? She's quite a character—wrote a very nice one in answer to their request. She sent it home and the folks get a kick out of it. Oh, how I hope they do their bit to make our dreams come true.

I've just been staring into space trying to find words to describe how I miss you and long to be with you. Ah, how great it is to be alive and in love with someone like you.

Goodnight, dearest,
Alice

OMAHA
Fri. night, Aug. 25
11:45

My darling:

I just told the night supervisor that I don't want to see her again tonight. But I just bet that something will come in pretty soon. Had quite a list of outpatients again today. Some of them are fun.

Dr. Lyman Heine was swell. He let me do the tonsillectomies & made the nurse the assistant. Then he sat down & said, "If you want any instrument—reach for it." Everything went swell, but I was surely glad that he was there when I hit a bleeder. There has been no hemorrhage since.

Why is it that after all of the departments give up on a case, they turn to ORL & say that there must be something in the sinuses? We have been getting such silly consultations recently.

Another intestinal obstruction is in tonight & I want to see the operation. The trouble with this hospital is that we know most every case that is in & I don't want to miss out on a single interesting case.

I wrote to Rochester again today, so our requests for a personal interview should come there together just like we will.

And about TB. Darling, I am afraid of it. We have had very little training in it, and I need more but am not too anxious to get more.

Please be careful.

You should have seen the children in pediatrics the other day when we brought a colored child in. We have no colored wards, so we put the kid in a cubicle alone & all the others formed a ring around & just looked. Quite a sight for some of these country children who have never seen a Negro.

Sweetheart, I am thinking of you and praying constantly that our trip is successful.

> Love,
> Joe

OMAHA
Monday night, Aug. 29
10:45

My darling Alice:

Two such sweet and lovely letters from you today. Dearest, I am the luckiest man in the world to have the love of such a wonderful girl like you. I envy these fellows here who can call up their fiancée every night—but even though you are so far away I feel so fortunate because I know that there is no other one like you anywhere.

It's 1,100 miles to the only girl for me—and soon she will be here. Although I cannot show you anything to compare to the Blue Hawaiian Room or Pontchartrain Beach or the dozens of other beautiful things that you have in N.O., we will go to the Bombay Room, Royal Grove at Peony Park, and the Paxton. Darling, I cannot express the pleasure it will be to have you here.

Two more days on admitting room. I did enjoy it even though it meant very little sleep.

Gee, you must get to see more patients in one week than I expect to see all year. Just absorb all of it because you will have to teach me an awful lot.

Have a chronic inflammation of the inner ear. I hope that we get to operate before I go off of service. I have only seen one other one so far this year

Dearest, it is a wonderful feeling to be in love with you.

Joe

1:40 a.m.

My darling:

Just got through with a hospital home delivery—2 senior students do it & I watch & give advice (believe it or not). Everything went OK and now I hope I can go to bed. Have another patient down with sodium amytal so expect no trouble.

The weather has changed—OBs are increasing.

Please forgive this short note. I just had to say that I love you dearly and am so anxious to have you near me. Now I'll catch up on 2 nights sleep, I hope, & have pleasant dreams of you.

Love,
Joe

New Orleans
Mon. nite, Aug. 29

My dearest one—

Dr. Fader surprised me today. He was watching me do a proctoscopic examination and he said, "Is that the way you're going to do it at Mayo's?" I answered that he shouldn't mention it as I was too afraid I wouldn't get to go. He said surely I would, and "So you don't want to stay here?" Then I told him that I had special reasons (and he didn't have to be told who the special reason was) for going to Mayo's. He said, "So Charity is second choice—Well, we'll keep you if you don't go up there." Then he gave me permission to check out the Sunday before my vacation so that I might get a head start. Gee, everyone is so good to me. I surely don't deserve it and can only hope that this good fortune continues.

I was up at 2, 4, and 7 to take the blood pressure of a peptic ulcer patient. Today it is gradually getting stronger and we have started him on milk and cream, one ounce of each every two hours. He says it surely tastes good. I wouldn't have thought of starting it so soon, but Dr. Hull says keeping the stomach empty doesn't help control the bleeding, and that fluids are needed. As you probably know, I believe anything he says is OK. But I still think our patient has pericardial effusion instead of pleural only, as Dr. Hull says.

My dear, I do so long to be with you—

All my love,
Alice

OMAHA
11:10 Wed. night, Aug. 31

My darling Alice:

I planned to go out tonight until one girl put a toy in her mouth and it stopped halfway down her esophagus. Gee, the way our Dr. J. H. Judd does those esophagoscopies, they seem so simple. Anyway, he recovered the toy. Now she can swallow and everyone is happy.

45 more minutes on admitting room—and I hope nothing else happens. Had a couple of tendons severed in a case this a.m., and was I glad a surgeon was in so he could do it.

I will carry two services, Gyn & ORL. The latter should not be too heavy & the laboratory will do most of the blood counts.

Everything is too quiet around here tonight. I just expect a call in a minute. Or probably another of the interns will come & break my neck for playing my radio so loudly. But truly when I write to you I forget everything else and have been guilty of having a roaring radio many times.

A chapter of St. Matthew & then dreams of you.

Goodnight, my love,

Joe

OMAHA

11:40 Sat. night, Sept. 3

My Beloved One:

Cedarblade left and handed me a ward full of OB patients. The resident and I made rounds. What a nice group of happy, contented mothers holding their precious babies closely. It is very pleasant work.

We broke a record this a.m.—16 minutes from the time the patient came to the hospital entrance to the time she was delivered with sterile drapes, etc. However, I did fear it might happen on the elevator.

Am getting caught up on Gyn. And now I have a new ORL patient. He'll have to wait until tomorrow.

Gee, another whole week of anticipation of your visit and our wonderful time together. Nothing else interests me now, darling, except you. I live to work for you & work to live up to your standards and ideals. Why, I can't even be cross because I wouldn't want you to hear.

And now, pleasant dreams come soon & don't be interrupted by a call from OB.

Love,

Joe

OMAHA
Tues Night, Sept. 6
10:10

My darling:

Another full day. The baby business is not rushing and am I thankful or I would never half keep up—in fact, I'm one physical &
2 blood counts behind now. But A.C. came back to town and I declared a vacation.

Gee, it was fun to sit & talk with him about Rochester. He got out of the hospital last week. We spent about 2 hours in the quarters just talking. Uncle Mac is the same radical fellow, talking about everything but pathology. A.C. agrees with me that McCarty is the most stimulating teacher that he has ever had. Darling, I enjoyed the evening thoroughly. Everything reminded me of you—from Dr. Adson's sarcastic remarks, Dr. Hench's clinics, the staff meeting and, of course, the Valencia. Van's dance band is still at the Pla-Mor—and apparently Rochester has two new nightclubs. We will make them all again.

Yes, the big tree is still on Silver Lake—too bad it isn't a live oak with Spanish moss hanging from its spreading boughs.

Darling, I am so anxious to dance again. It has been oh so long since we danced to "Harbor Lights" in Alexandria. And, better, just to sit and look into your eyes. It will be glorious.

I love you,
Joe

NEW ORLEANS

Fri. nite, Sept. 9

My dearest—

One more day and I can start on my much anticipated trip. I'm still afraid to get excited about it for fear something will happen yet. Gee, everyone wishing me luck and all—it's a grand feeling.

And today, each time I wrote 9/9/38 on a chart, I thought about it being your birthday—I insist that we have a chance to celebrate your birthday when I get there.

I'm afraid you are working too hard. It must be terrific to have two services, especially since you are on 24 hour duty in OB. Are you the only intern on OB? Gee, we have 6 or 8 this year. But I suppose you don't have a separate colored OB ward as we have.

Dr. Fader told me goodbye tonight and wished me a good time as he is going to take off the weekend to prepare for school. Next week the students start on the ward. I suppose we will really feel like big shots, what with assigning cases to them and checking over their histories and physicals.

Darling, I hated like the devil to miss being with you today, but my thoughts were.

I love you,

Alice

'How I hate to write this'

September–December 1938

———⟫●⟪———

Omaha
Sat. night, Sept. 17
11:10

My darling Alice:

Dearest, I never felt as lonely as I did when I saw you leave today. I watched the train go around the bend until even the smoke disappeared and my heart seemed to stop. My loved one was leaving, and I would not see her again for several months.

The past five days have been like a dream—something that I want to live & relive again. The clothes you wore, your smile, the way you combed your hair, the firm pressure of your hand, and the touch of your lips thrilled me and will live in my memory forever. Darling, I cannot tell you just how much I adore you & wish that you were here tonight. It is beyond my power of description, but suffice it to say that I want you above everything else in the world.

I have been receiving a lot of compliments about my Dr. Baker. Everyone thinks that you are grand—and do I know it. You are perfect.

I stopped to see A.C. at the Nu Sig house. Of course, he wanted to know why we didn't come by. And then he said, in his usual abrupt manner, "Joe, she is Plenty OK!" with emphasis. I had been telling him for a year, but now he knows for himself. Darling, you are wonderful. I'd give anything to be riding south on the same train with you tonight, dearest.

9 a.m. Sunday

What a night—got two seniors for the home delivery. After that
it seems that every OB in town came here. Had five patients in
4 hours. I stalled off a few with sodium amytal but I never saw a
busier place. I recall going to sleep at 4:30 & telling the nurse to call
at 5:30 but I awoke at 8. And believe it or not, Cedarblade is back—
that gives me only Gyn with 6 new cases to work up.

Darling, working hard is allowing me to forget the loneliness and
longing for you but, darling, my thoughts are always with you.

I was certain that I heard your beautiful voice several times last
night. If it only had been real—like the past five days. A true heaven
on earth.

Sweetest, I miss you more and more every minute. I love you,
Alice, and how I would like to whisper it into your ear.

Joe

NEW ORLEANS
Sun. nite, Sept. 18

My darling—

How very sweet and thoughtful of you to wire me. It made me feel
better to realize your thoughts were with me so. And oh, how I am
missing you.

I wanted to write you last night, but my pen gave out of ink on
my first page to Mother so I had to neglect you both until I could
get the pencil at Little Rock. I've just finished an 8-page letter to her
in which I tried—and utterly failed—to portray what a wonderful
time I have had. It was just perfect—and now I hope I can occupy
myself in reliving and re-appreciating each single moment of it
rather than thinking about how far away it all is and how I long to
be with you.

And I've been worrying about you! How did you possibly work last night and today? Gee, I slept until 10 o'clock this morning—and feel so guilty thinking how long you had been working.

Again, please take care of yourself—and here is a good-night kiss with my love—

Alice

OMAHA
10:45 Sunday night, Sept. 18

My darling Alice:

I am getting quite well caught up with my work—only one history & two physicals left for tomorrow. Believe it or not, all of the lab work is completed.

All of my patients wanted to know when you are coming back. They all were impressed by you. And how they would like you for their physician.

Called Dr. Stastny. She was sorry that we could not see her again. And she said, "Dr. Baker has a pleasing personality and will make a fine physician. Joe, you are lucky." She likes you very much and wants you to come back again.

Tomorrow school starts and dozens of students are coming up on the wards. They always manage to get in the interns' way—I know because I used to. And they really don't help any under the present system.

And now, memories of the past and high hopes and dreams for the future. I'll read the thirteenth chapter (should I say "our chapter") of Corinthians before I retire.

Darling, we have so much in common, think the same, do the same things, and have similar likes & dislikes. What else can anyone desire?

I love you,
Joe

NEW ORLEANS
Mon. nite, Sept. 19

My dearest one—

Thank goodness for a busy day, but in spite of that, I missed you so very, very much. Oh, what heaven it will be when we can be together.

Albritton really had a busy time. It seems the admissions are increasing markedly. The students are saving us a lot of work, though. I worked up 5 cases (briefly) this afternoon and am behind 3 or 4, but they are skin cases and can wait better than the medicine cases.

Everyone is asking about you and my trip. Gee, I can't begin to tell of the wonderful time I had. Gosh, being with you was the grandest and most wonderful of all.

And listen, darling I don't want you to change all of your plans because I said what I did at Mayo's about possibly practicing in New Orleans. I just said that because they asked me directly and—gee—I had no plans, but I had to say something, and that seemed to be the only thing I could say. But wherever you go and want to practice, I'd be proud and delighted if I could be included. I'm afraid the place wouldn't make much difference to me.

Do remember me to your folks. Gee, I love them and enjoyed being with them so much. Adela is marvelous and Dennis—well, he's just the cutest and smartest thing ever. I like Louis lots, too—well, I liked everything and everyone I saw in Clarkson. Oh, and do remember me to Dr. Stastny—Gee, I believe I'm more anxious to go back than ever.

But I'm most anxious to be with you again. Darling, I love you and miss you every minute—and please don't work too hard.

Love,
Alice

OMAHA

8:40 Tues. evening, Sept. 20

My darling one:

Imagine, I get to come to the quarters and relax in the evenings. But it gives me more time to think of you and realize just how much I really miss you. Dearest, it gets worse every hour. Only a week ago we were at home—what a pleasant evening, and such a memorable 4 days to follow. Yes, we are miles apart, but still I feel you near me all of the time. You are my inspiration and my all. How did I ever live without you?

One of my patients' husbands brought some pears, peaches & apples for us—so the interns will feast tonight & tomorrow.

Father is coming down for the new car tomorrow—Noma, as we now call it. I hope I can spend some time with him.

Cedarblade just came in—he would like to get a residency in Chicago. He said that this business of living apart from his fiancée was tough. And he had to tell me, just as if I did not know it.

Darling, we would certainly have an easier time to get into Mayo's if each of us had a year of residency. I'm not giving up hope but just wondering. Would it be possible for me to get into Charity? In Path, Surgery or Medicine. I see they take 4 residents in Path, 9 in Surgery & 8 in Medicine. Do they ever take anyone except one of their own interns? It would be nice to spend a year together there first, make our acquaintances with the staff & then go to Mayo's. Undoubtedly you could get into any service that you desire. In fact, I could make a personal application, too.

Don't misunderstand me. I am not discouraged about Mayo's, but I want to make certain that we will be together after next July, & I fear that my chances at Mayo's are not the best for one year. So just get me a little of the information, please, just in case we don't make it.

Darling, I really dreamt about you all last night. Here's hoping that pleasant experience is repeated very often. I miss you terribly.

Joe

New Orleans

Tues. nite, Sept. 20

My dearest—

My, but I enjoyed hearing from you today. Yesterday seemed so long without a letter from you. More than that I missed being with you, listening to your beloved voice—and feeling your arms around me. Ah, but I have such sweet memories now to live over and over again.

And you say that your heart stopped when you saw the train pull away. Darling, I could hardly stay on that train. Seeing you stand there and wanting so badly to be standing by you instead of leaving you for another 4 or 5 months—well, it was all I could do to sit still, and I just couldn't take my eyes away from you. Oh, how I long to be with you.

Business has quieted down somewhat, and the students are going to be a lot of help. We shall be interns at leisure compared with those of the U. of Neb., I expect. And please, don't you work too hard.

Every song makes your memory that much closer. Perhaps it is fortunate that "Harbor Lights" is not played so often now. It would be almost more than I could bear.

The war situation is still a scary one. The only outcome I can foresee is a gloomy one. I am hoping I am wrong. I just hope it doesn't mean much bloodshed.

And darling, I love you so very, very much.

Alice

NEW ORLEANS

Fri. nite, Sept. 23

My dearest—

This is really the life, having the students do all the work for you. I shall certainly hate to leave Medicine service especially since I hear that the students do not help with the charts on the Pediatrics ward. Dr. Fader was laughing today at how scared I had been the first day. He was certainly right—and now I dread leaving the service.

I shall certainly try to find out all I can about residencies. There are several interns in Path from other schools this year. In fact, all except Gretchen are from out of the state. However, Gretchen says that one must have the year as intern in pathology before he can get his residency. As to medicine, LSU has chiefly LSU graduates this year, but I have hopes that you may be able to get it. Also there is a rotating residency in which there is one out-of-state man now—I believe it is a 2-year residency. I'll also find out more about it. As to Surgery, they have chiefly out-of-state men. But both Medicine and Surgery are 3-year residencies. Would you want to sign up for that long?

Personally, I believe you'll get in Mayo's this year—and am positive you can get in next year, if not this one.

Dot and I used her brother's tickets for the Loyola-Springhill football game tonight. Gee, I never had such a good seat—on the 50 yard line. I've never seen so many fumbles in one game, but it was football and I enjoyed it. Loyola won 13–0. I see where Loyola plays Creighton on Nov. 13. It should be a pretty good match, but nothing like an LSU-Nebraska game would be!

I'm getting so many heart cases on my ward that I'm going murmurmad. And I still can't hear some of these diastolic murmurs even when they are described to me in detail. May I borrow your ears sometimes?

One of the boys has been asking several questions about applying at Mayo's. He pretends it's for someone else's info. But I imagine he is thinking of applying himself. I'm just hoping it won't hurt my chances. Selfish, am I not?

Darling, I miss you and long for you every moment, and am praying for the happy day when we can be together again. Until then—

> All my love to you,
> Alice

New Orleans
Sat. nite, Sept. 24

My dearest Joe—

Such upsets! Ole Miss is leading LSU by seven points. Alabama won over USC. Which just goes to show you, you can't tell. I surely hope LSU does something. Ole Miss is supposed to have only a fair team—but there goes another touchdown. No, just one yard to go for Ole Miss. It looks too bad for LSU.

Dr. Huff was so cocky about USC winning from Alabama that I bet him a quarter—and did I enjoy collecting it.

Gee, not one more touchdown but two more—20 to 0. Oh, boy, how that hurts.

I got another typhoid case tonight—at least, I think that is what it is. The other case, a typical case of typhoid clinically, with decrotic pulse and everything, has had negative cultures—blood, urine, and stool—as well as agglutination, so we must keep him on our ward instead of sending him to the contagious unit.

Darling, I feel as if part of myself is missing—for it does seem that life is complete only when we are together. It's a new feeling but a very dear one. It seems hard that we must be so far apart (in miles), but no one any nearer can ever fill your place.

God was good to me in letting me have your love. May it be His will that we may soon enjoy the realization of our dreams.

> All my love,
> Alice

OMAHA
Sunday night, Sept. 25
7:00

My dearest, sweetest Alice:

The Chase & Sanborn hour—I do hope that you are listening too. It is another one of our favorite programs.

Today has been a very easy day on the wards—no new patients. Cedarblade is checked out to me and even OB is slack. Maybe I am a jinx or something. I hope a couple come in before he returns.

Got to go to church today—and met Dr. & Mrs. W.L. Sucha. The Dr. is a surgeon on Creighton staff & a very good friend of mine. Had a nice time at their home and then made a call with him. Incidentally, they are going to New Orleans for the Creighton-Loyola game on Nov. 13th. They plan to go to Cuba but may have a few days stop in N.O. Of course, I told them all about you & you must meet them—and I'd like to have you get acquainted with them. They are about 45 years old and, unfortunately, have no children. Mrs. Sucha will be particularly glad to see you—and Dr., too. I would delight to go down with them but I'll wait for a better time.

How is Dot? I hope that she gets that X-ray residency. I know that she deserves it. And Frances? Give them all my regards.

I've got some more charts to finish tonight, but I'd rather have some OBs.

Football tickets will be out next week. I may get to go to the November games.

Dr. Sucha loaned me a book, "The Diary of a Country Priest." It promises to be good.

Darling, I'm hoping & praying that we will be together next year. So far our prayers have been more than answered.

Joe

NEW ORLEANS

Sun. nite, Sept. 25

My own darling—

News bulletins are very disturbing tonight. I wonder what the outcome will be. At least England and France are holding faith with Czechoslovakia—at least, to a greater extent than it would have seemed at first.

Today has been a slow day but tonight, when Bernes and another friend came to see me, I got a new case. He's in pretty bad shape and has enough physical findings and symptoms to equal those of three more usual cases. Another interesting problem for us.

And this weekend, I start Pediatrics. I'll surely have to do some studying before then. I shall be all out of practice on such patients. I also get newborn service. I think the newborns are the cutest and dearest of all babies. But I surely dread doing jugular punctures. I've done only one fontanelle puncture, but the jugular vein punctures look much worse.

Dot just came in. She has been playing bridge all afternoon and winning as usual. Now she's begging me to get her a Coca-Cola, so I don't know how much longer I'll get to write in peace. She says tell you "Hello" for her.

Well, the days are slowly passing and the time of your next visit is approaching. Thank goodness for that to look forward to. One of the boys sat down by me at dinner the other night with this greeting: "Don't you think she'll make a cute Yankee, Dot?"

All my love,

Alice

NEW ORLEANS
Mon. nite, Sept. 26

My own dearest one—

Payday again, so we had to celebrate. We went to see Dick Powell in "Cowboy from Brooklyn," and of all the goofy pictures, it certainly took the prize. It was so silly though that it was enjoyable, especially after listening to war news all day. Hitler made a very bragging talk, didn't he? I just wonder if a lot of it isn't fluff.

A German girl I know slightly went home for a week this summer and conditions there must be terrible—but they couldn't even express any criticism of Hitler in whispers. I think she was very glad to get back to the U.S.

Maude Bailey, the girl who takes care of our hair, said tonight that she was worried about her husband. He is at an army camp now, and on his way to promotion to a captain. Gee, I hope the reserves won't get a call, but I still think you were wise in joining the reserve. If war comes, draft will probably also soon be enforced, and the higher a commission you can get the better.

It all seems unreal, however. I could never speak so calmly about you going to fight if it did not seem an improbability.

God help us. May that never become a reality.

I love you darling,
Alice

New Orleans

Wed. nite, Sept. 28

My darling—

I went to see Dr. Grace Goldsmith today. We had a grand talk. She told me frankly that she had a very good friend on the medicine staff at Mayo who had a great deal to do with her getting a fellowship there. Also, he had to help her to get the department she wanted. She doesn't think I have nearly as good a chance of getting in Medicine as in OB and Gyn. Fortunately, I've always liked OB and Gyn, so I'll not mind changing too much.

Do you think we should postpone our applications another year though? I'll wait for your answer before I write to Mayo's. I don't think you'll have any difficulty at all in getting a residency here, especially since, with the new hospital, they will want many more residents than they've ever had before.

The Path sounds good. However, the year of internship which is necessary first includes bacteriology, serology, and a little true Pathology. If that is what you want, I don't think you'll have a bit of difficulty.

Well, Pediatrics service should be interesting. I think Albritton and I shall share the same wards again, but this time there will be half of 3 wards, rather than one. I suppose there won't be many more cases, though.

Darling, time is passing, even though it be slowly, and the time shall surely come when we shall be together then. Until then, my thoughts and dreams are of you.

Love,

Alice

Omaha

11:10 Thurs. night, Sept. 29

My adorable darling one:

What a heavenly day—made so by two letters from you. I read & re-read every word that you said—particularly plans for a vacation. I have asked for either late Dec. or Feb.—and the only problem now is will I apply at Charity next year. If I do, I would like to make a personal application—and when would be the most suitable time?

Dearest, again that brings up our plans for next year. I want so much to be near you.

Didn't you mention applying at Charity anyway? And failure of either of us at Mayo's would mean separation of from one to three years more, which would be unbearable. It might be advisable to take additional work so that the chances of failure would be less. I have sent for application blanks for Charity. I should like a year as path intern if possible.

It seems that I have been making the decision without consulting you. What do you think about it? Should we take our chances at Mayo's or take some work together elsewhere first? Above all, together is what counts.

The tensity of the war situation seems to be abating, which is very fortunate. I hope that they reach some sensible agreement without bloodshed. Although I will always feel that the Czechs were treated quite badly.

I have been looking for Little Jack Little tonight but was unable to find him. Perhaps he is not on every night, but I know he is playing at the Hawaiian Room and there is a special table waiting there for us.

Dearest, I miss you so very much, and I am constantly dreaming of the happy moments that we have spent together, and the heavenly days and years to come when we will be inseparable, professionally & socially. I am the luckiest man in the world to have your love, my wonderful one. And you have all of mine.

Joe

NEW ORLEANS
Thurs. nite, Sept. 29

My dearest—

What a grand letter from you today. And you too hear Little Jack Little broadcast from the Hawaiian Blue Room. Isn't his orchestra good? Perhaps we are listening to the same programs and are together in spirit, at least.

I was told to come to a meeting tomorrow. It seems that the Pediatrics Dept. wants to give us some instructions before we start. By the way, the head of the dept. is a very good friend of Ray's, and told him that if he could do anything for me he would be glad to. Would you be interested in a residency in Pediatrics? I'll bet you could get it. Also, I think there might be a very good chance of getting one in Medicine.

The European situation seems to be a little easier tonight. What do you think of the developments? Do you think Czechoslovakia is having to give up too much?

I am looking forward to meeting Dr. and Mrs. Sucha. I hope I can see the Creighton-Loyola game, too. Dot has tickets for tomorrow's Loyola-Birmingham game, but I'm wondering if I shouldn't stay in and try to brush up on some Pediatrics.

All my love,
Alice

NEW ORLEANS
Fri. night, Sept. 30

My darling—

I've been in one of those contrary moods all day, and now I'd like to crawl into your arms and have a good cry. You remember me telling you that Gretchen has developed a minimal pulmonary tuberculosis lesion, don't you? Well, she had another X-ray today, and there is a cavity about the size of a quarter. Poor kid, she's not saying a word—except that her biggest job is yet before her, that of telling her mother. She had been keeping it from her, but now she'll have to be told. She's the best sport about it I ever saw. She's whistling away right now.

Thank goodness I'm off the TB service now. Even though I know precautions are taken there more than elsewhere, I'm a big coward about it.

I have 2 wards on pediatrics which have been quarantined because of measles—that should give me a chance to catch on before I get very many admissions, I hope. I surely feel dumb about Pediatrics. And did I hate to leave Medicine. Sister Adele, the supervisor, told me goodbye and wished me well. She's very sweet and very competent. I'll just have to go back and follow up some of those cases.

Gamble had the service I take tomorrow and he showed me over the ward. He asked all about you and we had a good talk. Oh yes, Jernigan also has a minimal tuberculosis lesion and is out on bed rest. Nice conversation, eh what?

Darling, as always, I miss you and long to be with you—I feel so unworthy of your love.

Bless you, and I too am praying that we may be together soon—

Love,
Alice

OMAHA
Saturday night, Oct. 1
10:15

My own Alice:

The war news has reached a low ebb, and we can once more listen to programs without being interrupted by bulletins and flashes. But I don't agree with all of the decisions of the four powers in Munich, to open the Sudetenland to Hitler. It does save bloodshed, and apparently "might is right." Still—

About Mayo's. It is a very real problem. Undoubtedly, it is the best place to get training and the ideal place for both of us. And we both have as good a chance as any to get in. Although I have said that there is no word like failure, what would we do if they would hold off one or both of our acceptances? I could perhaps stay on here as instructor in anatomy, go into the Civilian Conservation Corps, or work with some M.D. in Omaha, which would make me very close to Rochester & you. April 1st is awfully late to obtain other residencies. What have you planned? Obviously, if we do go to Charity next year, it may mean that we stay there. The path residency does not sound so good. If we do plan to practice in N.O., it might be advisable to have a lot of contacts there. And the training there must be good.

But Mayo's is our dreamland. We met there, and so many of our most precious moments are interwoven with the clinic. It would be wonderful to spend three years there together. Are you willing to take the chance of possibly being separated for a year or without an appointment next year? This is the first time I have ever hesitated on taking a chance, but we cannot be discouraged by Dr. Balfour. There are still a few weeks time, and I'll be awaiting your reply.

Darling, I'll be praying daily that things will turn out in our favor, and I feel certain that they will.

I love you so much,
Joe

NEW ORLEANS
Sun. nite, Oct. 2

My dearest Joe—

Oh, what a long day Sunday is. I spent most of the day with my prematures. I'm taking the colored newborn service the first 2 weeks 'cause it's more work than the white, which I'll have the last two weeks. Admissions on my regular white Pediatrics ward have been very slow but will probably pick up when the quarantine is over. I have some cute little kids, but what I hate is having to take blood, etc. The poor kids cry so much and I feel for them.

I see that Lloyd C. Douglas has a new story running in the Cosmo-politan, "Disputed Passage." The ad for it says, "Is there room for love in a modern doctor's career?" I hope I know the answer to that—at least, for two young doctors in whom I am very interested—ahem.

Dr. Amédée Granger, our X-ray big shot, tells Gretchen that he doesn't believe she has a cavity, but that it is fibrosis resembling a cav-ity. Everyone else who has seen it thinks it's a cavity. She is going to bed anyway—for an indefinite period. She told her parents last night and they took it fine, of course. She is the best sport about it I ever saw, but I know it is worrying her lots. She's worked her way through school and deserves the breaks more than anyone I know, but she seems to be getting only the bad ones.

Dr. J.R. Schenken says he won't let her finish in Path, that the work is too hard. Maybe so, but I don't believe general internship would be any easier unless they purposely made it so.

Darling, I love you so and miss you so. It is such a joy to think of you and know you care for me. It drives away all my blues to dream of what we are looking forward to. I'm anxious to know if you think we should postpone our application for another year. If we try this year, I must write to Dr. Balfour and change to OB & Gyn. Oh, wouldn't it be great for us to be accepted, but career or not, for me the most impor-tant thing is being with you.

All of my love,
Alice

OMAHA
Monday night, Oct. 3
9:30

My sweet Alice:

What indescribable pleasure I derived from reading your two letters today—mingled only with the sadness of Gretchen's case. I do feel so sorry for her. I hope that she keeps up her courage and takes a rest. Hundreds of cavities have healed under the proper regimen. And, darling, I am so very glad that you are off TB service. I have been so worried that some of those patients might be a bit careless and cough, etc. And please still be careful, darling, and I'll be careful, too.

What a hot day we had—96° at 5 p.m., and it felt much worse. Oh, for some cool N.O. rains. Fortunately, we did have some cool weather when you were here, at least giving you the proper impression of the north. Yes, I am still telling everyone about the nice N.O. weather and how much I would like to be there with you.

Although we could not be together so much at Charity as at Mayo's, our chances to get in may be better there than at Mayo's. I feel that my chances are poor at the Clinic. What would you rather do? I still prefer medicine, but the more surgery I get to do, the better I like it. No matter what we take, we will always help each other.

So far I plan to come down at Christmas, but it is not definite. Even that will be awfully long to wait to see you. In the meantime, it might be advisable to change your application to OB & Gyn if you prefer it, & I am certain you will have a better chance if we decide to leave our applications for this year.

Darling, I miss you so very, very much.

Joe

New Orleans
Tues. night, Oct. 4

My dearest—

I'd give most anything to be with you right now, Gee, it's funny. I used to wonder about the love proposition. I never had felt like these people say they do when they fall in love. And I had decided it might be worth trying but had never found anyone I could become sufficiently interested in. But with Mayo's and meeting you—well, there was no trying about it, I just couldn't help myself. Darling, I'll never be able to understand how you chose me to make the happiest girl who ever lived, but I'll never cease giving thanks for it.

And now, darling, to try to be sensible. That is an awful job you gave me—to ask me if I'm willing to take a chance on being separated from you for another year, and darling, to make me completely satisfied about it, I want you to do just as you would do if you hadn't me to think about. I truly meant that when I told you that the last thing in the world that I want is the thought that I have interfered with your career. Darling, you have so much to offer the world. You will never be satisfied with anything mediocre and will always be on your toes with the best to offer at all times. Why, I would be miserable, feeling that I had done anything to interfere with that wonderful future of yours.

First, I would like to know if one refusal means more difficulty in getting in later—that is, at Mayo's, of course. If so, you will probably be right in wanting to wait for more preparation before you apply. However, for the life of me, I can't understand how you could fail to get your appointment. But you know Dr. Balfour's attitude toward you better than I, and you are the one to decide. It hurts to think of giving up a fellowship at Mayo's without even trying. Of course, we might feel better by not trying than we would if we got refused. But, there will be about 1,200 other disappointed ones who have tried and failed. We should be able to take it.

As for myself, I believe I have as good a chance now as I ever will. I can't change my sex (and I don't want to), which seemed to be their chief objection to me. You see, there's no redeeming feature for me—they'll just take me or leave me.

As for the thought of being separated from you another year—well, the thought is just about unbearable, and I just don't want to think about it. Dearest, surely some way will open for us, and I'm praying that it be the right way for both of us.

There's Little Jack Little playing "There's a Faraway Look in your Eyes." He must be playing it just for me. It's so true. I hope you are listening. Do write to me as frankly as I have, please. And all my love goes with you.

Alice

NEW ORLEANS
Wed. night, Oct. 5

My dearest Joe—

You should see my pet. She's a dwarfed child, apparently due to pituitary insufficiency. However, we're trying thyroid alone on her now. She is 7 years old and the cutest little thing. She has the biggest, most expressive brown eyes.

You should hear the children discussing me. They argue whether I'm a nurse or a doctor. One of them called me a lady doctor and was immediately called down by another who said I wasn't old enough to be a lady doctor but was a girl doctor. The older boys have a new name for me. It is Dr. Bakerman, and every time I pass by them they ask me for a loaf of bread—Ha. It's fun, even though it has its bad points.

I had real difficulty in getting a Wasserman from a 20 month old child today. She fought and screamed like a little tiger, and then crawled up into my arms and went to sleep. I don't see why she would do it since I was the one sticking her.

Mother wrote me that she had a nice letter from Dr. Joe. But she won't send it to me because she thinks (and rightly so) that I would keep it with mine. I prize every word that you write.

Darling, little room left but room to say the words I enjoy saying most—

All my love to you,
Alice

Omaha
Thursday night, Oct. 6
9:40

My darling Alice:

I often wonder just what this man Hitler will do with all of his illusions of conquest. I hope he remains on his side of the ocean. And 50 years from now we will look back at this time of the world's history.

However, in 50 years we will look back at the present time of our life as one marking only the beginning of our lifelong love for one another. It will grow deeper as the years go by, but I do wonder if that is possible, because my love for you is immeasurable now.

I realize, darling, that I have been stalling on this residency & fellowship business. Now I have received some information about Charity. I believe that you are right in saying that once accepted we could not change for the period of time for which we have a contract. In short, it means that if we go to Charity we forget Mayo's for several years or entirely.

I have thought & thought about this ever since you left, this business of residencies, and it has resolved itself into two possibilities.

If you don't mind, I will discuss them, and ask for your opinion and answers to the questions.

1. We stay at Charity (I mean you stay & presuming that I get a residency). What would you take? Or would you rather take your training elsewhere? This would mean that we would have to live apart in the hospital, but undoubtedly see each other very, very often for a period of 3–4 years. Then, if we wished to practice in N.O., our plans & contacts would be made. I would take surgery or medicine & make a personal application in Dec. This would mean that we would start immediately next July 1st—and be assured of a position next year (providing I get accepted & I know that you will).

There are advantages & disadvantages to the training there, but it must be one of the best places in the country, especially with "Charity The Beautiful." Of course, it does not have the prestige as Mayo's.

2. Our second possibility is to continue with our plans to Mayo's. Acceptance of both of us would be the realization of the greatest dreams possible. It would mean training under superior men &, of course, prestige. Of course, we could be together more than at Charity. However, there are several "ifs."

a. One or the other of us may not be accepted now or later. That would mean 3 years separation. If you get in & I don't, which will possibly happen, I could stay here another year. After that perhaps some residency in Minneapolis. If I get in & you don't— I could not ask you to stop your training to come there with me. Could you get a position close?

b. If neither of us gets accepted, what will we do next yr? As I have said, I could go C.C.C. or in anatomy here. It is much too late to get a good position then.

c. Finally, would getting rejected or postponing our applications have any effect upon our future standing there?

d. Salaries could be essentially the same considering maintenance at Charity. 3 & 4 years at Charity bring better monetary value. But money is of least importance.

Now, darling, in view of these facts—

1. Would you be content to stay at Charity?

2. Have you heard how good your chances are at Mayo's? Mine are average, according to Dr. Poynter. If we only would be certain of Mayo's, it would leave no doubt.

I think it all amounts to the fact that we want to be together as soon as possible & at a place where we can both follow our careers. My votes are cast for Charity. It would seem odd to destroy all of our carefully laid plans for Mayo's, but if we apply to Charity, our application to Mayo's can still be pending & if we fail at the first, we should get the second.

I imagine I have failed in expressing all of my views. It is a complicated problem—and I will be expecting your answers. Again, I will say I love you so dearly, my darling.

Goodnight,

Joe

NEW ORLEANS
Mon. night, Oct. 10

My dearest—

I've a feeling that this is going to be a very unsatisfactory letter. I've been trying to think straight all day, but everything just keeps going around in my mind. May I postpone serious discussion for a while? I'm tired tonight and my cerebration is nil. However, you are absolutely right, as far as I am concerned, about the question being chiefly that we may be together somewhere.

You make me very happy in your kind words about needing me. I assure you, though, that it is the other way around.

Dot is in one of her raving spells. Gee, I'm glad she is finding radiology so interesting. She is doing fine work and I think the staff men realize it. I don't think she'll have any trouble staying, but she may decide to go elsewhere. That is certainly a fine line that she is in. Her ambition since childhood has been to find a cure for cancer, and she's getting as near to that as anyone today.

By the way, it isn't that I mind staying at Charity. It is just that I was so full of dreams about Mayo's yet. I'd have to decide whether I should want a residency in Medicine or OB & Gyn. Tonight I'm even wondering if I could get a job as assistant teacher in anatomy. No doubt the review of the loss of so many prematures has its bearing on me feeling less clinically minded, and that no doubt will pass.

Darling, this much I do know. I hope with all my heart that we may be together next year and from then on. I'll try to write a more sensible letter tomorrow.

Goodnight, and all my love,
Alice

NEW ORLEANS
Tues. nite, Oct. 11

My dearest one—

Darling, you are really a sweetheart. I enjoyed your letter tremendously today—and am sorry I wrote such a tacky one last night. My only excuse is that I was dead tired. But I feel swell tonight. The only thing which could make me feel better would be to have you with me.

The chief objection that I find with this baby business is that everything happens at night. I went all day with practically nothing to do and then got a new case tonight. I don't believe I've had but one patient come in during the day and that was the diabetic, who has caused her share of night work. However, the service has been rather slow and I was glad to get a new patient tonight. And it promises to be a very interesting one. I'm expecting a positive Wasserman to explain a lot of it, but I may be wrong.

Now, to answer your questions. Of course I would be content to stay at Charity. Don't you know, darling, that the place would really make little difference as long as you were there? And I do think the training should be good here. I'm wondering if all my asking for recommendations from Mayo's would hinder my chance here. I think you should have little difficulty in getting in. I do hope that we won't have to accept anywhere else definitely until we hear from Mayo's. Do you think we could manage that way?

Just the thought of being with you next year gives me the most thrilling feeling. How inadequate words are to express it. But it is a delicious feeling which I shall continuously cherish.

> All my love,
> Alice

NEW ORLEANS
Wednesday night, Oct. 12

My dearest one—

The city is making big preparations for the Eucharistic Congress. Canal Street is waving with flags and banners, palm trees adorn all the lights (a new idea but quite effective), and other lights have the official emblem. They are expecting quite a crowd.

Frances is going to check out on me next week or the week after, so I'll be assured of getting off Christmas week. It will be perfect for you to come then—and it's only a little over two months off. Let's hope it passes quickly. I wish your folks could come, too. I'll bet they would enjoy our December weather. Oh, and will I enjoy it while you are here. It will probably rain continuously—but who cares?

We saw Bing Crosby in "Sing, You Sinners" tonight. It was a good picture and the "Small Fry" act was especially good. However, I like the song "A Pocketful of Dreams" best. It seems to have the effect of lessening any worries that one might have. Our pocketful of dreams include our future happiness, and we are truly fortunate to have a such a pocketful even if they are only dreams—as yet.

Isn't it funny. Although I've missed being with you ever since last August, I miss you more and more each day. My visit to the "info desk" at school and receipt of my precious letter are the bright spots of the day. If loving you at a distance of 1,103 miles fills my life with hitherto unknown joy, what will being near you and working with you mean? Darling, I am most fortunate and I love you dearly—

Alice

OMAHA
Wed. night, Oct. 19
11:00

My darling Alice:

Just in time to hear the Holy Hour for Men from New Orleans. Gee, I'd like to be at the Eucharistic Congress. It must be magnificent, particularly being in N.O. I am enjoying the description over the air—and how I'd like to see it with you, dear.

Dr. Drummond just called me again. It seems that he went to bed and now someone bolted & wired his door shut. And I can't help it if I found a wire & pliers and wired the door handle shut. Well, well, well—perhaps I'll let him out in the next hour.

And again to the radio—the Benediction must be beautiful—and with all of the candles lighted. Wouldn't television be nice. It must have been a very impressive ceremony. I hope to hear more tomorrow.

Attended medicine staff meeting tonight. Some of those fellows certainly like to razz each other.

Cedarblade is all excited—& rightfully so. Tomorrow his fiancée will be here. I am anxious to meet her, but I know that she cannot halfway compare with my Alice. Darling, I adore everything that you do—and how I cherish all of the letters from you—especially the first one 15 months ago. If time would only pass so that we could be together again. Since I have your love, darling, nothing else matters.

I love you,
Joe

NEW ORLEANS
Thurs., Oct. 20
1:30 a.m.

My dearest —

I've just returned from Midnight Mass. It was lovely. It was held in the new stadium at City Park—do your remember seeing it when you were here? I've never seen so many people, and when the lights were turned off after the people had lighted the candles, it was the loveliest sight imaginable. The altar was under a huge glass canopy of yellow and white. It was a beautiful ceremony, and all the while I felt you beside me. To know that you were worshiping with me and that this was your wonderful religion helped give it a greater significance to me. Dot's sister-in-law's uncle, a priest, went with us, and we felt quite conspicuous, being the only ladies among a huge number of priests.

Dot just said to tell you that you missed the most beautiful and impressive sight she had ever seen, and I fully agree with her. How I wish you might have been here.

Oh, but it won't be long until I can see my beloved. Oh, darling, I care for you so much it fills and overflows my being.

All my love to you,
Alice

OMAHA
8:10 Thursday night, Oct. 20

My dearest Alice:

Dearest, we have not said anything about residencies or fellowships for next year for some days. It is still a problem.

How would you like to go to Boston or New York if we don't make Mayo's? Drs. Stastny & Mildred Clark & several others from here were at New England Hospital for Women & Children & say the service is grand. Or how about Bellevue or some in New York? Some of the services start in July or October. Or Cleveland? I am writing for literature & blanks from several Boston & N.Y. hospitals. It wouldn't matter if we would not be in the same hospital—but that would be best. Dr. Stastny said she would write recommendations for you if you would desire. I have some very good friends at Long Island College. Just as long as we could get good training and be near each other. Would you consider going east? Perhaps you would like to get some training there, too. I could possibly get my pathology there. I will write for some applications & let you know. Personally, I feel that our chances at Mayo's would be better later—or perhaps we might stay elsewhere. I am wondering if you could not get a bigger volume of OB elsewhere. And medicine is good in the east. Or would you want to stay at Charity?

Above all, we want to be together next year and forever after, but also to complete our training. It will be grand to be practicing together, but now we want to get next year's plans settled. Would you care to investigate some of these other hospitals?

Just hearing news about some more possible wars in Europe— gosh, I wish they would settle it. Certainly heard a lot about it at home last weekend. There have been meetings of sympathizers around there for several weeks, & collections are sent to Prague. Lodges, clubs & religions of Clarkson & vicinity all have united in criticizing of the final decision. The papers are full of editorials, etc.

Heard Bing Crosby again tonight. How I would like to sit beside you & listen to it—and every other program. And now "Heart and Soul." Yes, darling, every love song makes me yearn for you more and more.

Goodnight, my dearest,
Joe

New Orleans
Mon. Nite, Oct. 24

My dearest—

What a day! My case of bronchopneumonia who was admitted last night turned out to have an acute abdomen. To make a long story short, they finally decided to operate on him tonight and found a ruptured left-sided appendix with pus-filled appendicitis. The appendix was very large, not walled off, and about to perforate again. It was removed and drains inserted, but I'm afraid his chances aren't so good. Gee, but it was a puzzling case. I believe it was a good thing they operated even if it had ruptured.

I hardly believe all the residencies are taken for Charity for 1939, for they'll need several more with the new hospital. It sounds interesting, this further work in the East—especially if some of them are open for October. That should give us time to hear from Mayo's before we have to answer them. Gee, I'd surely like to know our exact chances at Mayo's.

Darling, it makes no difference to me where we go if we can be together, but Mayo's still seems like the land of dreams come true. But you are the essential part of all my dreams.

Alice

My dearest—

Today has surely been a full one. I started out scrubbing for an empyema aspiration. The patient was admitted on my service and Dr. J.A. D'Anna, one of the most prominent surgeons in N.O., saw him there before he was transferred to his service. So he always calls me when he does anything. His idea is to try to get the chest completely free of pus by aspiration only. My confreres (ahem!), the Pediatric staff men, seem to think he's all off, but if it will save open thoracotomy, it might be worth it. At least, I'm trying to keep an open mind (another ahem). And I enjoyed scrubbing (even though I did fear all the skin was coming off from the stiff brush).

Do you realize, that is the first time I've ever scrubbed at Charity? Again I'm thankful to Dr. Jones for the experience he gave me at the Veterans Hospital 3 summers ago. Next year I get my surgical half of my internship.

Darling, I miss you so much that it seems I can hardly bear it. Just think, though, two months from tonight, we'll be in Alex again. Happy will be beside himself at feeling his new master at the wheel, but the other person on the front seat—well, she'll be in seventh heaven. No, it will be in fourth heaven, won't it?

Goodnight, sweetheart,
Alice

NEW ORLEANS
Wed. Nite, Oct. 26

My darling—

I'm now waiting for a blood-matching report. My resident decided to give a blood transfusion to one of my prematures who is in very bad shape. We'd better hurry and get the report or the baby may die before he gets the transfusion. I wonder if the work on the baby isn't severe enough to offset the good done by the transfusion, but I suppose I shouldn't have such thoughts. Thank goodness the resident is the one to attempt the transfusion. I know I could never hit such small veins.

I had fairly good results with tetrachloroethylene on a little girl with tapeworm infestation. The result is an 87-inch worm. However, I'm not sure the head has passed yet. Do you get much experience with tapeworms up there? This is the first case I've handled myself.

Poor Gretchen. Her latest X-ray shows a slight decrease in the size of the cavity but a marked increase in the amount of infiltration around the cavity, plus a beginning lesion (infiltrative) in the opposite lung. They told her only that the cavity was smaller. I surely feel for her, but she is still taking it like the swell sport she is.

Later

There was the blood matching report. All three waiting mothers were compatible. But just when I got back to the nursery with the blood, Dr. Rena Crawford said, "I think the baby is dead." We used the resuscitation for about 30 minutes and caffeine into the heart, but it didn't work. Gee, there are certainly a small percentage of prematures who survive here.

Dr. L.J. Kleinsasser, Tulane's surgical resident from Nebraska, finally approves of our weather. He says he feels much more energetic, and his smile has been much broader since our cold weather has begun. I think our opinion of him increases even more with continued acquaintance.

But the Nebraskan I long to see is far away—in miles, but not in spirit—for he has a special place in my heart.

All my love,
Alice

NEW ORLEANS
Fri. Nite, Oct. 28

My dearest—

Mother came in this evening. I was so very glad to see her. It has been so long since I saw her last. That was on my way to Omaha, you know, and so much has happened since. It is past midnight now, but I've an idea we haven't nearly stopped talking yet.

You should have heard Catherine, the little pituitary dwarf I wrote you about. Today she climbed up on the desk where I was writing night orders and said, "Dr. Baker, I love you with all my heart, my liver, and my stomach." Now how do you like that for a declaration of love!

Mother says to tell you that she is scolding me for being up too late. But don't worry, it's her fault. I have to stop and talk between each line or two. And tomorrow we'll stay in and have another talk fest—all the boys on the floor want to go to the football game. I just hope my work stays as easy as it is now.

Well, I found my first malaria parasites yesterday, started quinine, and you should see the fever curve flatten out. It really gives one a thrill to see some results. On the medicine ward, we had so many patients that as soon as the diagnosis was made, we gave the patients prescriptions and discharged them.

I've also come to the conclusion that the majority of treatment in pediatrics is rest in bed and watchful waiting. These kids just naturally cure themselves.

Darling, we have talked of nothing since Mother came except Joe and the Holoubeks. And how I love to talk about you all and have Mother join in with praise of you. Meantime I am missing you more than ever, and wishing you were with us.

All of my love,
Alice

OMAHA
Monday night, Oct. 31
9:10

My own darling:

Your letters were quite an inspiration again today—especially tonight. OB has been unusually heavy and I need "shut-eye," but after reading your letters, I am ready for another night. Gosh, what would your presence here do? It would be all that I ask for, and it would stimulate me to conquer any difficulty.

The "Carnation Contented Hour" is dedicated to New Orleans tonight. His description of the French Quarter, Cabildo, Pontalba, St. Louis Cathedral & Jackson Square brings back so many treasured memories. And now about Canal Street. I have never been so fascinated & attracted by any city—all because of you, my darling. So much romance there with you. But it will not be long until we can be there together.

Gee, I'll hate to leave OB. It seems that I have grown very fond of Wards E & F. And especially when I've gotten to do episiotomies. I was proud of the one this p.m.—20 minutes to repair it. However, I did a tenth day examination on one that I would rather not claim. She will have a large scar. But pediatrics should be interesting. They have a lot of cases in at present.

I see Catherine is giving me some competition. You are so adorable—no wonder she likes you.

I love you so much—an old statement, but coming from the bottom of my heart.

Joe

NEW ORLEANS
Monday, Oct. 31

My own darling—

How I enjoy Mondays—two letters from my beloved. And how I treasure each word. Dr. Huff told me today that I might check out to him Christmas week, so things are really looking rosy. I was so glad I found out before Mother left for she had been worrying so about it. Now she went home happy in the thought that we—you and I— would be home for Christmas Eve and Christmas. If you plan to arrive in Alex on Christmas Eve, I'll probably also leave then and get in about 7:30. Then I can check out beginning Christmas Day and have 5 whole days off.

I think you had better bring a heavy overcoat, for although the thermometer doesn't go so low, people from the North say they get just as cold or even colder than they do at home. It seems to be the humidity. Could that be right, professor? Anyway, you'll probably get to see some more freak weather.

I'm dreaming of the day when you shall be practicing as you want to practice medicine and, I hope, I can be assisting you. It's a precious dream, for my love is all yours—

Alice

NEW ORLEANS
Tuesday, Nov. 1

My darling—

What a nice thing for state holidays to happen occasionally. It gave me a chance to work up 4 patients I had inherited, read over the others' charts, and try to review a little ENT therapy. I hope to be a little better prepared for clinic. However, our course in EENT was very negligible and I dread the first few days.

Darling, I have a confederate in my insistence that you take your fellowship at Mayo's—which I still can't honestly understand why you shouldn't get. Mother agrees that you must take that opportunity. That prestige will be to your advantage during all your years of practice

Darling, I could never forgive myself if you gave up your chance at Mayo's because of me.

Why, while you're up there, I may even get in somewhere or somehow at Alex and get to be with my folks. It would be darned hard, but I would truly be more satisfied.

Darling, I'm trying to say that I love you very, very dearly but never want my love to stand in your way. Oh, dearest, let's let time help us decide. I can't bear to think about it too much. May the Lord help us and show us the right way.

Here is a goodnight kiss and all my love for my sweetheart—

Alice

OMAHA
Thursday a.m., Nov. 3
2:30

My darling Alice:

And I thought that Pediatrics was an easy service. Well, I was fooled—and waded knee-deep in a group of very acute cases. What diagnostic problems some of them are. Have an acrodynia that has been here for 3 months. Have only one diabetic and she should be dismissed soon. Yes, I had a death the first day. An 8 yr. old boy had appendiceal perforation 2 days before admission & he has been kept alive with transfusion & intravenous fluids for 1 week— and he had to die my first day on. Just now a case came in as acute osteomyelitis and I think it's Rheumatic fever. Certainly run into some diagnostic problems as compared to OB. There, one glance usually was sufficient.

We had our own Halloween celebration—did everything but put on sheets & tour the wards. The best was stuffing a bed with pillows in ward L and placing artificial brains for the head and then telling the night supervisor to come see her new patient. Her hair has come down from the standing position by now.

It's late but still time to say that I miss you terribly and I know that everything will turn out for the best for both of us. I love you so.

Joe

OMAHA
Sunday night, Nov. 6
11:45

My own darling Alice:

We had snow this morning, and most of the ground is still covered with a layer of flakes. It's just the beginning of winter and I have decided that I prefer the South.

Had Ped staff rounds this a.m. The thing I enjoyed was the staff having "fried Henske pride" for breakfast. Every time Dr. J.A. Henske said something, they all seemed to line up against him. And I am getting tired of his "When I was in Vienna." I'm surely glad he is only a visiting man & not on regular service now.

Do I get an earful of rales. So many children have a tracheobronchitis (so they call it—just plain beginning pneumonia to me). As you say, we let them get well themselves with O2 & steam as an aid.

Next Sunday I'll be listening to the Creighton-Loyola game—will you be there? I'll visit Dr. & Mrs. Sucha before they go. I want them to come to see you—and if you have the time, could you please take them around the hospital? Oh, how I wish that I could go too— but darling, it will be only about 46 more days and I can hold you tightly again.

My dearest Alice, I adore you and always will.

Joe

OMAHA
Wednesday, Nov. 9
8:45

My sweetest Alice:

Another long dreary day without you—enlightened only by your delightful letter. Darling, I don't know what I would do if I would not receive your letter just one single day. They are the joy of my life.

Did a lot of reading today. Of course, the 13th chapter of 1st Corinthians and then the Sermon on the Mount in Chapter 6 of St. Luke. I never realized so much truth could be found in one chapter. The theme of "Magnificent Obsession" is there.

Ah, Kay is on now—I'll have to turn my radio low so that I would not disturb everyone. Gee, it would be fun to dance to him with you in my arms. I bet my ankles will be stiff in December. That will be over 3 months without dancing again. Here he comes with "So Help Me." Oh, darling, I wish I could sing these songs to you under a magnolia tree or a live oak covered with Spanish moss, anywhere, my dear, even on the plains of Nebraska—or someday in Mayo Park.

Darling, as a woman you have 1 chance in 4 to get in at Mayo's. I have about 100 in about 1200, but we have made our applications and let us try it. The good Lord will show us the proper way, I am sure. Something will happen and we are certain to be together always.

Joe

Omaha
Thurs. afternoon, Nov. 10
4:20

My darling one:

First, I love you a thousand times more than I can ever state. You are wonderful and I want you to be mine always. Now, what I wanted to tell you but didn't want to worry you.

I had a cut on my left forefinger, which I received from a cart. I enlarged it, let it bleed, put alcohol on & disinfected it thoroughly. Sunday night it became tender. Monday I soaked it three times & most of the night. I have been in the hospital since then, under observation, with hot packs & sulfanilamide. White count 12,800. I feel swell except a bit dizzy from the prontylin.

There is only one thing that I need—and that is to have my private physician here. Darling, if you had been here I am certain that I would be well already. I am to be dismissed in the a.m.

Darling, I hope that you do not mind that I did not tell you before, but I did not think it would last this long & I did not want you to worry about it. Please don't, dearest. I am getting as good care as I can be without you being here. Hot packs every ½ hr, dry heat, sulfanilamide 60 grains per day, limit fluids, bed rest—radio, books & my daily letters from you.

But this hospital life is not like intern life. Gosh, the beds are hard.

The interns are cheerful souls. They come in with stories of fellows with strep infection that—well, they don't finish. One of them, Donald Ross, just came in with a bouquet of white carnations and set them in my drinking glass. I wonder where he swiped them. And now the supervisor of nurses & her stooge. I wish those supervisors would stay out of here.

My gosh, here they come to change the sheets or something again. I'll be so glad when tomorrow comes around.

Darling, please excuse this poor penmanship. It's worse than usual, but I've got a hot pack on my left arm & am not supposed to move it. And please don't worry. I'll be out tomorrow.

Darling, I love you & I'll take care of myself for you.

Joe

OMAHA
Friday, Nov. 11
9:00

My darling Alice:

There is no peace in this hospital. If it is not a visitor, it is a nurse with a hot pack or hot water bottle, a supervisor or somebody else. Now, I finally got rid of everyone and am listening to Guy Lombardo.

Got 40 rads from radiology through three ports to my left hand and arm this p.m., and the lymphangitis has cleared up. What does Dot think of X-ray therapy for strep? I think it is swell if it works. My nodes are not half as tender, blood count has gone down, and I should be able to get up tomorrow for sure. No temperature, etc., and it is awfully tough to stay in bed—particularly on such hard mattresses.

The assistant supt. of the hospital came up to see me today, and I told him that I have started to follow all of the radio serials and won't be worth anything for work—as if I ever was.

Dr. Henske, the ped prof, called tonight and informed the telephone operator that I must get certain X-ray plates down to clinic in the a.m. Hot dog, won't he steam & spout if I won't get out & they won't be there.

Gee, I'd better get out quickly. I came down for one day and now it's for four. I owe money for stamps, newspapers, gum, etc.—and I am one of the fellows who should work while the others go to the game tomorrow.

I have had more time to sleep & read & think than I recall having had for ages. However, my sleep has been interrupted every half hour by a hot pack—and some of them are hot. Have read most of Washington Irving's works, but I have read very little medicine. In fact, I have forgotten about it entirely except that constant question "When can I get up?"

I have had so much time to think primarily about us—you and I. What the future holds in store for us we do not know, but we do want to be together.

I imagine that I messed things up rather badly a few weeks ago when I decided on someplace else besides Mayo's. It was a constant source of worry for me for some time, and if I upset you, I am sorry. Our applications are set for Mayo's. Let us stick to them and some way, somehow, the Lord will bring us together. I know that He will. We both have faith in Him, and He will not fail us.

So unless something unforeseen happens, we will leave everything as it is until April 1, and the Lord of all be with us then.

And please darling, don't worry about my hand. I just have a good case of internitis now & don't want to go back to work—ha.

> Darling, I love you,
> Joe

OMAHA
Sat. evening, Nov. 12
6:00 p.m.

My adorable darling Alice:

Here I am again—propped up with a little more freedom of motion, and I don't for the world of me see why I could not work today. But the doctor said another day. He said I'd enjoy the Pitt game as well in here as in my room. I got 40 rads through 3 ports again today & am to get another treatment sometime tonight. They use the portable outfit. Ever since we started it, the lymphangitis has decreased, believe it or not. Leucocyte count is down to 8,500 this a.m., so I am definitely on the way out tomorrow.

I have been listening to one of my prematures crying in the room above me for 5 days now—that's long enough. He must need a change of formula or something.

My "pal" Henske announced to the entire junior class that the Ped. intern is ill. The nut. I didn't want anyone much to know & now it will go like wild fire. If there is any thing I hate, it is having people come in and pity me. As long as they don't feel sorry for me, everything is OK.

I forgot to tell you that Father & Mother, Adela & Louis came to town last Thursday & were ushered up to my room. Were they surprised! I explained everything, & Mother said that she knew that sometime they would catch me in bed. But worst of all, in the p.m. when they were visiting again, a gray-haired supervisor walked in and found a new red streak & decided to call the intern. Well, I had to do some tall explaining to Mother again. Will phone tonight.

Later

Another hot pack—and again I reread your most enjoyable letters. I treasure them more and more. I look a sight—a hot water bottle is acting as a paper holder.

Just fixed one of the supervisors by putting ink on my bandage, & she thought I had gotten gangrene. Hot dog. Guess I'll pull a feigned faint on her the next time she sticks her nose in here.

One thing I have against this ward—it's too darned quiet. I'm used to noise—and lots of it. Four years in the Nu Sig house initiated me to that.

Talked to Dr. Poynter & he said that my chances are better than average at Mayo's. Dr. Charles Baker (pathologist from Methodist Hospital) was here yesterday, & he said I had a good chance of getting in this year & if not, for sure next year. That is all I know. But darling, why worry—but gosh, I do, too. If you want X-ray you might get it at Mayo's—or have you changed to OB? However, we must still realize that the competition is the greatest there (that is probably why we want to go). Let us wait until next April & then if we fail we can make other plans, OK?

Darling, I'm off to dream of you again, my dearest. And please don't worry. I shall be on the wards busy working tomorrow.

Goodnight, my love,
Joe

NEW ORLEANS
Sun. Nite, Nov. 13

My dearest—

I had a fine afternoon, but not perfect because you were not there. We saw Creighton lick the socks off Loyola. It was funny. I'd try to rant for Loyola, and then the thought that those big huskies on the other team were from Omaha just got me, and I'd find myself yelling at the top of my voice for Creighton—much to Dot's chagrin.

I picked out Dr. Sucha when I first sat down (since we were using Dr. Mattingly's tickets, we had a front row seat on the 50 yard line)—and sure enough, one of the players was soon hurt, and he turned out to be the doctor. No doubt I'm prejudiced, but I just naturally like the looks of these Northern men. He is fine looking—and apparently very interested in football. Dot and I got quite a kick from watching him yelling instructions to the players. It was a rough game and there were several injuries. I believe Creighton received most of them, but that may be because they were more active. I'll bet the Creighton men really felt the heat this afternoon. It was as warm as a day in July for the first half of the game and almost uncomfortable. For the third quarter it became very cloudy and caused apprehension among the crowd—and for the fourth quarter it was quite cool and nice.

Oh, yes, there was a touchdown made in the last three minutes of the game, just like a movie, except that Creighton, already 28 points ahead, was the one to make it. Oh, those Yankees!

Ah, another day during which most of my time was spent missing you—to be truthful, all of the time for you are always with me. Ah, 42 days from now will surely find one happy person!

Good night, dearest one,
Alice

OMAHA
Monday night, Nov. 14
9:00

My dearest Alice:

I finally was dismissed this a.m. feeling fine & dandy—but that didn't last long. I mean, 1 week in the hospital made me a little weak, & I had pediatric dispensary all alone & loaded with patients. But with a couple hours sleep I am feeling OK. Yes, not even strep can bother me much. Don't worry, I am watching my blood picture very carefully.

10:20

Darling, I'm in a daze. It's wonderful, perfect to talk to you, to hear your heavenly voice. That same thrill that I feel whenever I hear your voice, but magnified a thousand times by your presence near me. And to think that the time will come when I will feel that way all of the time. And let us hope and pray it is not far away.

And please don't worry, Alice dear. Yes, I'm still taking prontylin. I am OK now. Your call has been the best medicine I have had.

All my love,
Joe

NEW ORLEANS
Mon. Nite, Nov. 14

Dearest Joe—

I'm sorry I was such a sap as to call you tonight. When I got your second letter today and found that they hadn't let you out of the hospital as you thought they would, and that they were giving you X-ray therapy, I let my imagination run wild. I was so relieved when the intern who answered said that you had checked out, but couldn't resist the temptation to talk to you later when I had the chance.

Dot says tell you we enjoyed hearing from you and are glad to know that you are better. And while she is here to dictate to me, she wants to know if they repeated the X-ray therapy. She believes in 35 rads every other day for three treatments (if necessary) through as many ports as necessary, never exceeding four at one time. She says there is a great controversy as to dosages for infection, and this is her idea. I think she knows what she is about.

Dr. Sucha is going to come by the hospital in the morning, either before or after I have my clinic hours. He seems to be especially interested in orthopedics. He told me he was born near your birthplace, but several years previously. I'm surely anxious to meet him.

Darling, please forgive me for being such a pest. I hope that you are all well by the time this letter reaches you.

All my love,
Alice

OMAHA

Tuesday night, Nov. 15

9 p.m.

My sweetest Alice:

I am still dreaming of the voice that I heard last night. I never dreamed that anyone could thrill me so very much as you have whenever I hear you, my dear.

Started work this a.m. Got in a premature. Everything else was quiet, & about the time I started to get acquainted with the new patients, Dr. McLaughlin came up and in a quiet but firm voice said, "Holoubek, is this taking things easy?" So now I am to spend 2 days resting in the quarters. My gosh. So here I am, reading Life and everything I can get my hands on. But most of all I am thinking of you and dreaming of the time that we will be together. I'll wear out your letters & pictures pretty soon, but the memories are more vivid every day.

Dearest, I am counting the days until I can whisper soft words to you. Please don't worry your pretty head about my hand. It's all well & cured, but a doctor always tells his patients "to take things easy a few days."

Darling, I love you,

Joe

NEW ORLEANS

Tues. Nite, Nov. 15

My precious one—

I had an enjoyable evening with friends of yours—oh, I like Dr. and Mrs. Sucha so much. Why is it all the Northern people I meet seem so very nice—much nicer than most of these Southerners. Don't you suppose the climate has something to do with it?

And, darling, do they like you! It thrilled me so to hear them say so many nice things about you. I always knew you were wonderful, but it makes me so proud to hear someone else brag on you. Oh, I don't deserve my good fortune. How can you care for a nincompoop like me—but please don't stop. I would be absolutely lost without you, and your letters are my mainstay. Oh, how I hope our dreams come true.

Please tell me truthfully—and in detail—how you are getting along. I hope those X-ray treatments are as good as Dot thinks they are.

I love you,

Alice

Omaha
Wed. night, Nov. 16
10:00

My adorable darling:

I just missed Kay Kyser's program, but I went down to the general staff meeting this evening. It was limited to the discussion of cancer. It seems that the types that we get here are usually of the higher grades and very malignant.

Yes, I am still "canned up" in the quarters—reading & thinking & sleeping. One of the Nu Sigs brought me George Eliot's "Middlemarch," and from what I have read of it, she must have been a very brilliant woman.

My leucocyte count is back to 7500 again, so I'll go to work tomorrow a.m. I have been getting accustomed to using two hands again after having one in hot packs for several days. I became very right-handed. But everything is back to normal except my hair. Gee, it is long enough to curl. Three weeks without a haircut is too much.

I am glad you enjoyed the game last Sunday. And by now you have undoubtedly met the Suchas. Whenever I meet him he talks of football—either this fall's games, next year's outlook or spring practice, depending on the season. The last time I saw him, he had his car filled with boxes of "dextrin" which he feeds his men before each game. The energy may not be all due to meteorological stimulation.

I can't resist just sitting & dreaming as I hear the number "My Own." Just a few more weeks and we can listen to it together. Now for some sleep—it is all I have done, but tomorrow I start work. And don't worry—I won't do any work that I won't have to.

Goodnight, sweetheart,
Joe

OMAHA
Thu. Night, Nov. 17
10:30

My sweetest one:

Well, I got back on duty today. According to Dr. Charles McLaughlin's orders, only part-time work for 2 days, but the service is light and I am not attending dispensary.

Now that it is all over I believe that it was more serious than I had thought. I considered it as a joke until I started work 2 days ago and welcomed more rest. It is the first time any infection had weakened me so, but now I am back to normal. So I was told to quit "racing my motor" for a few days—well, I'll show them some first-class idling. I firmly believe that the 40 rads through 4 ports in 3 treatments at 24-hour intervals did more to help me than anything else.

There goes that number again—"Heart and Soul." It seems that whenever I write to you, some orchestra plays it. Wonderful.

Father and Mother came down to the auto show today, and I got to spend my usual few minutes with them. Noma looks grand, but she is complete only when you are behind the wheel.

Don't worry about me anymore because I am back on duty & feeling fine. But I still need your advice. Quick—a prescription containing you for that feeling in my heart.

I love you,
Joe

New Orleans
Thurs. Nite, Nov. 17

My darling—

I'm just getting more glad all the time that I called you Mon. nite. I know I couldn't have slept well for worrying—it takes so darned long to get mail from Nebraska. Now I can see you saying to yourself that you won't tell me next time, but please don't do that.

As the days pass, I see myself changing so much that I have to laugh at myself. I never used to believe that I could care for anyone so much that they would be in my thoughts continuously, and that just a word from them could make me the happiest person living. But it has come true. I'm absolutely a hopeless case—about you, darling.

I've just witnessed my first struggle between life and death. In all the other deaths I've witnessed, there has been no struggle—just the peaceful passing of a patient who has been waiting for death as a kindly visitor. But this was a beautiful child of about 9 years of age who was burned (2nd degree) over the whole right half of chest, right arm, parts of face, end of nose, and even the tonsils and pharynx. She was very restless and delirious before death and then, with a sudden shudder, she died. It surely was pitiful to see.

And now, goodnight, dearest. I sincerely hope you are getting a strong upper hold on those strep by now.

Good night, beloved,
Alice

CLARKSON
2 a.m., Thursday, Nov. 24

My darling Alice:

Dearest, it is empty without you here. The memories of your visit here are more vivid than ever—I do wish that we can repeat that soon.

Father & Mother are well and send you their love. Mother's sinuses have not been bothering her recently. And I got to drive Noma—gee, she is a dream—and all ours. The heater certainly comes in handy to melt the frost off the windshield. Yes, it is very chilly way up north now.

I didn't come home with A.C. as I had planned but took the 11:30 p.m. train to Schuyler & my folks met me there. My plans were changed by the pneumonia that came in. It happened to be the infant of a good friend of mine from Leigh (6 miles west of Clarkson). He had a temperature of 106° for 3 hours and was in profound dehydration. Stayed up most of the night with him. In the a.m. he developed convulsions. This p.m. when A.C. left, the kid was still plenty sick and I did not want to leave. Well, he looked a lot better tonight, so I took the night train.

The Union Station brought back pleasant memories again of you. And then there was that track on which the train left over 2 months ago carrying my beloved away from me. This yearning for you is increasing every minute.

Gosh, today is Thanksgiving. I have been so very fortunate this year, darling, so much to be heartily thankful for—my parents, and everything at home, and you and your love. That is the most treasured possession that I can ever have. Ours is not the "ordinary love." It is something so superior, so deep and beautiful, it can be considered sacred. Oh, dearest, I am so very thankful.

Time, please pass rapidly while we are apart and stop when we are together.

Now for some rest in my real soft bed and dreams of you.

All my love, Joe

NEW ORLEANS

Thanksgiving Night

My sweetheart—

Thanksgiving, our true American holiday, and one of the best. I spent it all alone today, for Dot spent the day with relatives. But I had such pleasant thoughts and dreams of future Thanksgivings when I hope to be very far from being alone, for I hope to be with the one I love.

I just called Mother. She asked me if I'd like to have some of the family turkey. You can imagine my answer. We had turkey today here at the hospital, too, but it certainly didn't taste like home. And were we surprised when they brought each of us a glass of wine. It didn't taste so good to me (but then I'm not a connoisseur at such things). But we drank a very appropriate toast at the table that we are all where we want to be next year. Oh, darling, next year—

Dot's aunt sent me 4 big pieces of cake, and I'm sitting here making a pig of myself. Thanksgiving is one day when that seems to be excusable.

Brrr—you should see your Sunny South now. A temperature below 40° is predicted for tonight, and our radiator isn't working. I called the engineer tonight, and, in a polite way, he insinuated that I must be slightly crazy, that the radiator was on. May be, but I'm sitting 3 feet from it and with my sweater on and am not comfortably warm yet. I'm afraid the room we bragged about being so cool during the summer is going to be rather cool this winter, also.

Tonight I have a special prayer of Thanksgiving. My most humble and grateful thanks to the dear Lord for my love.

Darling, you are the inspiration of my life—

All of my love,

Alice

NEW ORLEANS
Sat. nite, Nov. 26

My darling—

Frances has just come in and kept us in an uproar for the last half hour telling us about her trip to New York. She had only 3 days and 2 nights there but she must have made the most of it. She saw several plays, visited Bellevue Hospital, and went to the International Casino. She also bumped into Jack Dempsey when her train lunched. Quite thrilling. But most impressive seems to have been the snow. She says on the trip up the leaves were still on the trees, and on the way back they were covered with snow. She stopped at Philadelphia to see a friend of ours who is interning there, and altho they gave themselves 1½ hours to get back to the train, they got snowbound and barely made it.

Oh, it reminds me of my trip, but hers couldn't have been 1/10 as much fun for she didn't have your companionship to share.

The school had a holiday today—and I didn't get your letter. It will be terrible to have to go two days without hearing from you, but the thought of three coming in on Monday will sustain me, I suppose. With Frances back and the ward (ENT) quiet, I think I'll take some time off tomorrow. I can't realize the week passed so rapidly. I hear that the service I go to next—colored female genito-urinary at Pythian—has only 6 patients on the ward now. I can hardly believe it. I really like to have a little more to do than that.

Darling, I love you and miss you so. One month from tonight will find me so happy. Until then, dreams of that time must suffice.

All my love,
Alice

OMAHA
Monday night, Nov. 28

My adorable Alice:

It was perfect this morning, receiving three letters from you—every one so sweet, so much like a part of you. I have read and reread them—and every time I get more lonely and miss you more. Yes, we do have so very much to be thankful for every hour of the day—the fact that we have each other. Everyday is a day of thanksgiving and also a prayer for the realization of our desires and dreams. And I heartily join in your Thanksgiving toast, my dear. Let us hope that it does come true.

I go on Neurology, Neurosurgery, Psychiatry & Ophthalmology next month. Not that I will particularly enjoy any of them. I must confess that I do like pediatrics immensely, probably because there are so many diagnostic problems—and histories frequently inadequate. Had a laugh on the admitting room today. They admitted a patient with a diagnosis of "crying baby." I decided that it was nothing but a spoiled kid with no disease.

Kay Kyser—the same theme song that we heard that enchanting night in Alexandria. And to realize that similar nights are less than one month away. Again and again, from the bottom of my heart—

I love you,
Joe

Tues, Nov. 29

Darling one—

I feel as if I have been on a vacation. I took the afternoon off and spent it being most frivolous. Bernes was with me for a while, and we had lots of fun window shopping and such. There is nothing I enjoy more than buying Christmas gifts—if I have some money. But someway I can't seem to save much money on my huge salary. I'm afraid I'm going to have a tough time choosing gifts this year with so little time.

Did I wish for you this afternoon! Bernes and I went to Solaris, a large special fancy grocery store in the French Quarter, and ate oysters on the half shell and drank beer. It was fun but would have been so much more so with you there with us. Darling, how I miss you.

Dr. Val H. Fuchs, the chief of ENT in graduate school, gave us a very good talk on what the general practitioner should know in that line. He promises to give us notes with prescriptions, etc. I surely hope he does for he gave us some very interesting facts.

In twenty-six more days, I'll be perfectly happy, for I'll be with the one I love dearly.

Alice

OMAHA
Wed. night, Nov. 30
11:35

My darling one:

Abe Lyman just played "My Reverie." Dearest, how lonely I am.
The transmission of sound over those awful 1,103 miles is instan-
taneous—if only we could travel that rapidly. But I am always
with you in my thoughts. Now, "You're the Only Star in My Blue
Heaven." My greatest fortune was the day that I met you and then
our falling in love.

Gee, I hated to leave that Pedy ward. I have liked that service
much better than any other. Maybe it is because I like children so
very much. The cutest patient is a petit mal case, controlled by diet.
One of my staff men believes that idiopathic epilepsy in childhood
is comparable to diabetes—it can be controlled by diet. I took him
off the high fat diet today to see what will happen.

Darling, the days are so long without you near me. With Kay
Kyser's program tonight I could not help but dream of that eventful
day last June. Meeting you and your mother at Campti, the drive to
Alex, your home, your father, the wonderful dinner. The drive to
the magnolia trees, the park, and that night—how wonderful, the
moon and us. Dearest, I cherish those memories of joyous moments
forever. But soon all the time will be like that.

I love you,
Joe

NEW ORLEANS
Wed. night November 30

My dearest—

Well, my ENT days are over. I hear that I have 10 patients now on my new ward. I got a letter from Mother today. She enclosed a letter from Ray's wife, Marie. She sent a picture of herself and she looks quite fat—she weighs 110 pounds, and used to weigh 98–100 at the most. She is allowed to go out from the TB sanitarium once in a while, so apparently she is doing fairly well, although she complains because they won't tell her anything about her condition.

Mother is talking about Christmas. Gee, we're all so thrilled about it. We always have our family tree on Christmas Eve, and it's the most precious time of all the year to me. And this year, well, I never would have dreamed of more happiness than we are planning. Let us pray nothing happens.

I guess I did my last tonsillectomy today. One side gave trouble but the Beck snare cleaned out the other one fine. And for a change, today's listing of interns who had delinquent charts in the record room didn't have my name on it. However, I'm expecting a new crop to sign out soon. One of the Pediatrics wards is again quarantined, due to measles. Poor kids.

Darling, tomorrow means December, which means just 24 days more until I can see my beloved. How anxious I am for the time to pass quickly until we can be together.

All my love,
Alice

NEW ORLEANS
Thurs. night, Dec. 1

My beloved—

I wonder if you have been thinking of me tonight as I have of you. If there is anything to mental telepathy, you should have. Such dreams and hopes and desires in the air must produce some sort of waves or bumps or something.

Bernes and I had one of our good long talks tonight. And, of course, our hopes and plans for the future were uppermost. Sometimes it almost stuns me, the thought of how very fortunate I am. God has certainly been good to me. I've never had any hard knocks, any severe discouragement—and now that my life may be truly full and that I may truly live in the greatest sense of the word, I have met and, inevitably, loved you.

Darling, my cup is overflowing.

I feel almost ashamed to be praying for more—but surely, with all this, it is meant that we may be together. How I hope and pray that this may be so.

There is a notice posted downstairs that applications for residencies here must be in by Dec. 15, or they will not be considered. I can't help but believe that we are doing right in waiting on Mayo's. To accept a residency from here must mean signing a contract of 3–4 years, and it can't be broken by accepting elsewhere. I believe we are doing right to wait, but I want to be sure that you feel that way, too.

My service at Pythian is turning out to be very nice. My only objection so far is that I don't know what I'll do with the time on my hands. I have only 9 patients—can you imagine such a lazy girl as I shall be after a month on such a service? However, Dot and I started a French course offered here by a WPA teacher and it may help keep us busy. Anything to make time pass more quickly until Dec. 24. After I meet you, it may stop completely.

All of my love,
Alice

OMAHA

Fri. night, Dec. 2

My sweetest Alice:

I just spent a most wonderful evening with the Suchas. It was
the first time since their return that I had a long talk with them.
And how they enjoyed visiting with you. Their compliments were
endless—"She is such a sweet girl." "What a wonderful doctor she
is." "She is a perfect lady"—and hundreds of others. Of course, I
echoed and re-echoed them. Oh, dearest, how lucky I am to have
such a sweet girl like you fall in love with me. They enjoyed their
trip through Charity, the dinner & evening visit with you. Mrs.
Sucha said she would write to you this Sunday.

Was Dr. Sucha proud of his Creighton team! I think the 10
grains of sodium chloride before the game & at the half & dextrin
in tea may have helped to keep up their resistance. It must have
been a hot day.

It was so much fun talking about the places where we had been
together. My memories have made me lonely for those times again.
Finally Mrs. Sucha passed pralines. How well I remember the trip to
the Gulf and my first taste of them. Canal Street, Cabildo, St. Louis
Cathedral, Charity & Blue Room were all part of the conversation,
but best of all was news from you. Nothing else mattered. Gosh, you
must be busy, dear, with all the work they describe. I hope you take
it easy on G.U. now.

I adore you,

Joe

OMAHA
Sunday night, Dec. 4
10:45

My darling Alice:

I'm on Ward L giving a transfusion to the brain tumor case that we did this a.m. (and p.m.). My gosh, but she is restless—and the blood is going in much too slowly. And I wish she would breathe better, too.

What a day. Not that I don't like neuro-surgery, but it is rather tedious. The operation lasted until 2:30 and we were all rather tired by then. I do admire Dr. Keegan's calmness—very little conversation during the entire procedure. When something happens he says "o-o-ouch"—but he did let out a few damns. No one got bawled out—and it was all so different as compared to Dr. Adson.

Gee, this did not even seem like Sunday. It seems ages since I went to church this a.m. And was it cold walking back. That was one time that coffee did taste good for breakfast. It rained, snowed & turned to sleet this p.m. Typical Nebraska weather. Much too stimulating—and unhealthy, too.

I am taking on Pedy for Dr. Herbert Modlin for one week starting tomorrow. He will work for me when I am gone for my most perfect vacation with you.

Dr. Albert Broders will speak on carcinoma at the Methodist staff meeting on Tuesday. I hope I can attend. I think we both missed a lot by not getting acquainted with him better at Mayo's, but I don't think his philosophy can surpass Uncle Mac's.

Thank goodness—the last 10 cc have gone in. Blood pressure 110/75, pulse regular. Now for something to eat & finish my letter in my room.

11:45

Just found out that there is an acute abdomen due here from Clarkson now—so I want to see it.

Darling, you are my only inspiration. Everything I do is because of and for you. I cannot wait to see you again. The long-awaited December is here, and Christmas just 3 weeks away.

My dearest, I will always love you more than anything in the world. You are my everything.

Joe

Omaha

11:15 Tue. Night, Dec. 6

My adorable one:

Another pneumonia just came in. Gosh, these kids can get sick in no time. Fortunately, most of them get well as fast even if left alone. Had an interesting case on eye tonight—perforated cornea 3 days ago, but we are not worried about sympathetic ophthalmia—he had the other eye removed 20 years ago.

Had a very interesting evening—went to hear Dr. Broders. I liked his presentation very much, and he stressed the point that cancer is a recessive Mendelian character. I met him after the talk. He is a very interesting person, and I am sorry that we did not have more work under him. But perhaps we may sometime. All they had to do was mention Mayo's and the majority of physicians turned out.

After that I stopped at the fraternity house. A quite typical group—seniors playing bridge, juniors asking about patients, sophs arguing about the CO_2 tension in the respiratory center in a mythical case of an individual gasping for breath, and the freshmen worrying about the relationships of the Axillary artery & nerves in the first, second & 3rd division.

Then back to the hospital and we had a round table discussion about the impractical things we have to learn in medical school—such as the nitrogen content of guinea pig blood and others. Now with Abe Lyman, I'm "deep in a dream of you," and with your lovely letters—read & reread.

I am so anxious for the Christmas Eve at your home with you and your parents. It will be perfect.

I love you,
Joe

ALEXANDRIA
Wed. nite, Dec. 7

My darling—

Dearest, you don't know how I hate to write this. And please, promise me not to worry, for it's nothing and I promise to take care of myself.

Yesterday I had a slight pain in my chest, which got a little worse when I took a deep breath or coughed. So, old neurotic me, I got scared and had an X-ray plate made. Well, I have a very small area of infiltration in the right first interspace at the periphery. It's not even as large as a quarter. It is well circumscribed and everyone agrees that 4–6 weeks will cure it completely.

Naturally the first thing that came to my mind was to go home. Dr. Weilbaecher didn't want me to at first, but when I explained that Dad was a doctor and had specialized in tuberculosis, he agreed that was the best thing for me to do. Soooooo, here I am. Department chair Dr. George Bel gave me 4 weeks leave of absence. I feel very good, I haven't lost any weight—I haven't even had any fever, not even after the trip home today. So dearest, you see, it isn't anything to worry about.

They say it is the earliest case they've ever seen at Charity, and Dad says he's not a bit worried. He swears I'll be completely well in one month. And gosh, I feel perfectly well now.

And darling, if you would rather wait until next year sometime for your vacation leave, it is perfectly alright with me. I'm afraid we couldn't run around much for I'm going to stay strictly in bed for one month anyway. I have too much to live for to fool around with halfway measures. I aim to get completely well.

Ah, darling how fortunate I am to have had the plate made when I did. Believe me, darling, it's such a little area, it's almost foolish to take it seriously.

Oh, darling, I do love you so. I don't want to be the cause of your worrying. Please don't, for I'm not.

All of my love,
Alice

OMAHA
Sat. Night, Dec. 10
9:30

My adorable one:

Darling, I don't know how to start, except to say that I was very shocked to learn the news this morning. I had never dreamed that tuberculosis would ever strike someone so very near & dear to me.

But I am so very thankful that you had the chest ray taken at the first sign of any symptoms. And, frankly, I would be very worried, but since you are under the care of your very competent father, I feel at ease. I have so much faith in him.

I am so very glad that the lesion is well circumscribed. A short period of rest and it will be well healed. And I know, darling—for your sake, my sake, and for our future—you will do everything to get a complete cure. Please don't get back to work too soon.

I promise not to worry too much but please keep me informed.

Darling, let us not feel depressed because of your illness. It is another of the obstacles that we have to overcome—and in years to come we will look back at all of this and thank God that we overcame them all. Only I wish that it would be me who would be sick instead.

Now, dearest, read a lot of books so that you could tell me all about them. But best of all, get a lot of good rest. I think you have been working too hard.

Now for my nightly reading in the Bible, a peek down at the wards again—and then dreams of you.

I love you,
Joe

ALEXANDRIA
Sun. nite, Dec. 11

My darling—

I had the greatest and nicest surprise this morning—the loveliest bouquet of flowers. It is so nice of you and I really am proud of them. They are lovely and they make the room look so cheerful.

I'm about to die of impatience. I want to hear from you again. But I shall get letters tomorrow and how I'm looking forward to them.

Alice

ALEXANDRIA
Tues. nite, Dec. 13

My own darling—

I wish I could halfway express to you how much your letter meant to me today. I have been awaiting it oh so anxiously, and how much better I feel now.

Darling, please do not worry. I almost feel ashamed of myself to be lying up here in bed, feeling perfectly well, with no fever or anything wrong that can be seen or felt, at least—and have Mother waiting on me and people being so nice.

Truthfully I'd be strongly tempted not to stay in bed if I hadn't these dreams of our future—dreams in which an old chronic TB cannot be included.

Soooooo, if bed rest and good care will do it, I'll get rid of it as soon as possible.

I've slept most of this first week and am feeling so rested and so good now. I guess I was more tired than I thought I was.

I'm glad you don't have any TB patients—but do you ever get them with some other disease, too? And although this may sound funny now, please do take care of yourself.

Darling, there's just one thing more. I'd love so very much to see you, but I'll still be piled up in bed and you wouldn't have much enjoyment for your Christmas holidays. And I know your folks will miss you terribly. Oh, I don't know how to say it—I do so want to see you, be with you, and go everywhere with you. But if you think it best to wait, truly I'll understand.

Dot has written almost every day, and Gretchen promises to write. I didn't even tell them goodbye. I was too anxious to get home.

Darling, the posies are lovely and the dreams they call to mind every time I glance at them—which is all day long—are lovelier yet. Bless you, my dearest. Even over 1,103 miles, your healing influence is great.

All my love,
Alice

OMAHA
Wed. night, Dec. 14
10:05

My adorable one:

This has been a rather slow day—and I am thankful because of the rather busy night on OB.

The Nu Sigs are having a Tom & Jerry party next Friday afternoon. It is an annual affair before Christmas and I hope I can attend—although I am not too crazy about Tom & Jerry drinks—but it will be fun to get together with the boys again.

Darling, it is only 10 days until Christmas. I am so anxious to see you. But tell me, dear, would the excitement be too much for you? I want to see you so badly, but yet I don't want to make you more ill. Of course, you will have to stay in bed and we could spend long hours visiting, without a care in the world. So unless I hear from you to the contrary, I'll arrive the evening of the 24th. I want to spend a happy Christmas with you & your parents.

I love you,
Joe

ALEXANDRIA
Fri. nite, Dec. 16

Dearest Joe—

Listening to Guy Lombardo and thinking of you—perfect enjoyment! Won't we enjoy listening to him together?

So you are still relieving on OB. I surely hope I get back to work in time to get OB and Gyn. I won't mind missing surgery so much—and I may not have to miss much of that.

Dot gave me some good news. She was asking her boss, Dr. James Barrett Irwin, why she had never before seen the plate of a lesion like mine. He answered that it was because they were hardly ever diagnosed that early and gave her an excellent research reference from which she prognosticates that there should be no activity after 2 months. She has certainly proven her friendship.

I have truly been lazy today. I've been reading some very light books, but none so far worth mentioning. It seems the local library has very few new books, and those it has are out. However, the librarian from the hospital is going to bring me some from there.

As you see, I have no news. Just the same old story, but how precious to me—

I love you,
Alice

ALEXANDRIA
Mon. nite, Dec. 19

Dearest Joe—

I believe you will be leaving Thurs. nite or Fri a.m., and this is the last letter until I see you. Oh, how happy that makes me.

The music over the radio is beautiful now. So many Christmas carols. Did you hear Lionel Barrymore read "The Christmas Carol"?

I have been receiving so many nice letters and gifts. It keeps me busy acknowledging them—that and my reading.

I'm listening to Eddie Cantor via Lincoln tonight. I can't seem to find Omaha. Probably you can find it when you come.

I see that Buddy Rogers is to be at the Blue Room over the holidays. Well, we can be much more comfortable listening to him from home, I guess (sour grapes). But I'm really going to enjoy these holidays so much. I'm sorry we can't do the things we had planned—but there will always be other times, and for you to be here will make my Christmas blissfully happy. I still thrill to the sound of your voice as I hear it in memory. Oh, how wonderful it will be when you are actually here.

I'm hoping that the weather will continue as warm and nice as it is now. And now, goodnight, but for only a short time—

All my love,
Alice

Omaha
Tue. Night, Dec. 20

My darling Alice:

Another day has passed—and only a few more until I can see you. How anxious I am for that time.

I started to town this p.m. and expected warm weather—but, on the contrary, it was quite cold. And what a crowd downtown—I finally ended up buying some Christmas cards and going home.

I am getting all of my consultations written up tonight so I will have all of my work done by then. I may have to help on receiving room tomorrow & Thu. since another intern is leaving, too. I hope the work is light now.

Gee, I see the AMA got in trouble in Washington. Not that we feel particularly sorry for Dr. Morris Fishbein. But I am not in favor of state control of medicine.

Went to the bus & train ticket offices today. Bus leaves 8 a.m. Friday & arrives 9:10 Saturday night. I cannot get such good connections by train.

Darling, how can I wait until next Saturday night when I will see you. And then for days we will be together—how perfect.

I love you,
Joe

'Darling, please don't worry'

January–March 1939

———>◦<———

Little Rock, Arkansas
Sunday, Jan. 1

Sweetheart:

The train is a little late. I hope you excuse the stationery but it is all I have for the present. Gosh, it was so hard to leave Alex. It seems I have left the most important part of me behind. Anywhere that I go without you, dearest, I find a strange emptiness. The solution, obviously, is to be with you.

I dread getting upon that train because it will carry me farther & farther away from you. I have had such a perfect time. This has been the loveliest Christmas that I have ever had, to say nothing of the most perfect present—you. Everyone has been so lovely to me in Alex. I enjoyed every minute of it.

Darling, you looked beautiful—especially at dinner today. I never ever wanted to leave you.

It's about train time—I love you, darling, and I miss you so much.

Joe

ALEXANDRIA

Sun. night, Jan. 1

My darling—

Dorothy Lamour is singing "Two Sleepy People" and, oh, how I love you, darling—and I guess that song was appropriate for the grandest week I've ever had. I certainly never thought I could enjoy a week in bed, much less enjoy it more than any time I've ever spent.

Oh, my. Now Nelson Eddy is singing "O Promise Me." It almost hurts me inside somewhere because it is so pretty, and it makes me long for you and for your arms to be about me. My dearest, I just can't write sensibly while he's singing that—

And now I'll try to do better. Mother says to tell you that although the night is beautiful and the moonlight lovely—why that should be, I can't imagine—the fluid in the barometer is trying to run out of the spout. So no doubt we'll have a storm before morning.

I'm anxious to hear from you. When do you relieve in Ophthalmology service? I'm going to feel much better about you now that you're not going to work so hard.

Darling, I love you—yes, again.

> Goodnight, my sweetheart,
> Alice

ON THE TRAIN

1:30 Mon., Jan. 2

My sweetheart:

Two more hours & we will reach Kansas City. No snow as yet and the sun is becoming almost unbearably hot as it shines in through the window—and to pull the shade down makes it too dark.

4:30 Kansas City

My letter was interrupted by an acquaintance with the dean of the Kansas State Graduate College. We discussed everything from politics to medicine. And then he asked, "What do you think of women in medicine?" "I am going to marry one!" Then I proceeded to tell all about you & how highly I regarded women in the medical profession.

All during the rest of the trip, my mind kept wandering to sunny La. to 1733 White Street, to the most adorable girl in the land. Darling, I can picture you now—reclining in bed, looking so fresh and neat, with your ever-present smile.

Sweetheart, my own dear sweetheart, I will see your face before me always. Last September I thought it was not possible that I could ever miss you more—but, darling, I was wrong. It was nothing compared to my desire to be with you now, the yearning for the touch of your hand, the warmth of your breath, and the touch of your lips. The sound of your sweet voice is all that my ears want to hear. It is such a difficult job to resist the temptation of jumping upon every southbound train.

I was so surprised at the warm weather here—very comfortable without a topcoat. Apparently the temperature went down to zero a few days back, but no snow as yet. Stimulating temperature—zero one day & 60° the next. I prefer the South.

I dream of you always—and I remember most vividly the picture of you as you sat at dinner yesterday. So lovely & adorable.

I love you,

Joe

OMAHA
Monday, Jan. 2
10:15

Sweetheart:

Arrived at 8:30—and I never hated to come to Omaha as much as I did now. And I was minus my black suitcase again, but it should come by the next train.

Called home & got to speak to both Mother & Father. It surely felt good, & all I talked about was you & your parents. They promised to come down soon & I'll talk to my heart's content.

If we could but relive the past week now—and, oh, darling, we will, and never be separated for a day.

What a perfect time I had this vacation—and all because of you & your lovely parents. My folks send their love.

Sweetheart, I love you,
Joe

ALEXANDRIA
Mon. nite, Jan. 2

My darling—

The red roses are beautiful. I love to smell them and look at them—so all but one are by the window where they make the most lovely bouquet. One beautiful bud is on my radio table where I can smell it. But I care most of all for the words on the card.

I slept most of the morning—in fact, I refused to be awakened, for I had nothing special to look forward to as I had last week, darling. So this afternoon and evening I read a book and wrote a couple of letters.

Daddy went fishing today and came back in seventh heaven. He caught over thirty fish and most of them were good-sized. So he distributed them to the Tysons and to friends at the hospital. Those we kept will be consumed tomorrow night in Dr. Jones' company, we hope. Ah, if it could only be like the dinner this summer with you and your mother and dad.

Mother and I played Chinese checkers tonight. She beat me so badly I wouldn't let her stop until I finally won a game and, at that, I won it only by one point. I believe I do better when I don't concentrate on the game, as I didn't when we were playing.

My ring is so lovely and a joy because of the memory of Christmas Eve—and the rest of the week.

My dear, I love you so very, very much—and I pray that I may be partially worthy of your love.

Alice

Omaha
Tue. Night, Jan. 3
9:00

My sweetheart:

Now I realize that the rumor about Urology & Orthopedics is correct—"You are one week behind before you start." So what—too much work to catch up, so why try. Since I promised to work less, I'll quit at a respectable time. The work is not too strenuous as yet, and I won't let it get that way.

Dearest, do you believe that I have gained 5 lbs.—I am up to 162 now. Several individuals remarked how much better I look. It must be the good Southern cooking with 8 days of seeing your cheerful smile. And perhaps less worry about your condition.

Received my suitcase this a.m. All intact, but suits slightly crushed.

Dearest, I feel out of place in my uniform again—and my stethoscope is always in my way.

Darling, how I wish that we could turn back time at least one week, so that I could spend those delightfully enjoyable days with you again. My heart aches for your presence. I want you near me all of the time.

Give my regards to your father & mother. They were so lovely to me.

Now to dreamland and you—I love you, sweetheart.

Joe

ALEXANDRIA
Friday nite, Jan. 6

My darling—

So your work is going to be hard, as usual. I surely hope it doesn't become too strenuous. Have you had a chest plate made yet?

Mother is so tickled about your gain in weight. She's been bragging about it—it's the best way to please her. She says you had better not lose it now, that it is to be stored up and increased on your next visit.

Oh, my dearest, I do miss you terribly. I can hardly talk about you and yet I do talk about you constantly. I have always known I could never love anyone without respecting him, but to have found anyone so perfect in every way—in ideals, training, native intelligence, and lovable personality. How fortunate I am. And I love you—heart and soul.

Alice

OMAHA

Tuesday, Jan. 10

My darling, [Dictated, nurse's handwriting]

You may find this script much more legible than mine. To make a long story short, I'm in the hospital again for observation, but not for what you expect.

I had acute sore throat this morning with no other symptoms. At about 10 a.m. I developed a rash over my face, chest, and back which blanched upon pressure. There was a greyish coating on my tongue. My temperature was 99.4. I was placed in the hospital with a diagnosis of, as you know by the history of findings, scarlet fever. Otherwise I feel very well, having no nausea, vomiting, or loss of appetite, and am certain that it is just a transient allergic phenomenon.

Darling, please don't worry because I'm under good supervision and promise to stay in bed all the time. It won't be necessary to call because I'm in isolation.

I didn't like urology and orthopedics anyway, so I decided I needed a rest. Perhaps it was my vacation that made me a trifle lazy. I assure you that I had sufficient sleep and rest the past three weeks and see no reason why this should be scarlatina. However, if it is like the present epidemic, it is very mild and doesn't result in complications.

As you expect, I'm letting my folks know before they find out by some roundabout untrue method.

I'll try to write a letter every day, but as you notice I have to dictate them because of isolation.

I'm sure I'd get well much sooner if you were here. Truly I don't feel ill and would be willing to go fishing, but the superintendent thinks it's advisable to keep me in, and furthermore I can't let you have more of a vacation than I do.

Love,

Joe

P.S. Please be careful of my last letter. It was mailed three hours before appearance of the rash.

OMAHA

Wednesday, Jan. 11

My darling, [Dictated, another nurse's handwriting]

As you see, I'm still in isolation. My throat's still red & my skin a little flushed. The diagnosis of scarlatina has been confirmed. My temperature varies from 99° to 101°, but I feel very well.

The Supt. of the hospital just came in & informed me that I'm to be transferred to the City Isolation Hospital for about a week. After that I'll probably get to go home for a week or two. The only thing I miss here is my radio.

Had a very comfortable night & truly, dear, there is no cause for worry. I'll probably gain some more weight because I feel so well.

The only thing that bothers me is the fact that I'll leave some poor intern my urology & ortho service.

Aren't we fortunate that I got my vacation previous to my present illness? In fact, we have been extremely fortunate, so much so that any transient illness is of no concern.

I hope to get a radio installed so I might get Kay Kyser tonight—primarily because you'll be listening & because the program brings back refreshing memories.

Please don't worry because, as you well know, scarlatina is very mild & develops no complications if properly handled. Furthermore my resistance is very high at present. But I would appreciate some of Mother's special cooking.

My address for the time being is City Isolation Hospital.

I love you, sweetheart—

Joe

CITY ISOLATION HOSPITAL

Thursday, Jan. 12

My Darling: [Typewritten]

I'm still blushing—and we thought it was just a womanly attribute. But I feel well. My temperature is down to 100.2. Throat only slightly sore and a fair appetite. As you would suggest, I am getting hot gargles, oil rubs, and bed rest. I am receiving 5 grains Acetyl Sal. every 3 hrs. No, I have not received antitoxin because the disease is unusually mild and it is unnecessary. Truly, dear, if this is as bad as Scarlet Fever is, I have no complaints. The only thing that bothers me is the strict isolation. My father and mother came to town yesterday, but after they found out that I was not very ill, they went home.

Incidentally, I requested that the fact that I am ill not be sent up north, and Dr. Francis Bean, assistant superintendent, said that recommendations had been sent already. Therefore I am certain yours had been mailed, too.

Of course, I am listening to Baby Snooks and Bing Crosby. I heard the play "Stella Dallas." What pleasant memories it brought back of Louisiana. And wasn't Kay good last night?

Please, Dear, you now know this is not serious and gives me a good rest for medical and surgical services. I am so anxious for tomorrow's letter.

I love you,

Joe

CITY ISOLATION HOSPITAL

Friday, Jan. 13

My darling: [Typewritten]

I finally have had my mail forwarded here from University Hospital. Your letters, now more than ever, make the days more bearable.

Dearest, I am getting well unbelievably fast. My rash is fading, face starting to desquamate, temperature 99.8, and I am eating my meals. Physically I feel well—except some generalized itching. I have had gallons of water.

I will not do any studying during this vacation. I fear it would weaken my eyes—or perhaps that is my excuse for laziness. Nevertheless, I won't read.

You won't like this, dear, but I'm growing a beard. My face was too tender to shave the past few days. And frankly, I look worse than usual. It is blond on the top lip and chin and black elsewhere. The radio programs tonight do not sound half as good as they did two weeks ago. Guess why?

I love you,

Joe

CITY ISOLATION HOSPITAL

Saturday, Jan. 14

My Darling: [Typewritten]

Another long day—but made very happy by your beautiful bouquet of flowers. They fill my room with a delightful fragrance. My staff physician, Dr. E. J. Kirk, admired them, too. You recall that we met him while waiting to see the Dean last Sept. He is going down to N.O. for some meeting this March and promised to visit you. There may be more Omaha M.D.'s asking you to show them through Charity at that time.

I just received your special delivery letter. That makes the day complete.

In case you are interested—my temperature has been normal all day. Now I have 15 days of quarantine left with nothing to do but be lazy. Rash is practically gone.

Talked to A.C. through a window today. He is a great pal. Here comes the "Hit Parade."

Give my regards to your parents.

> I adore you,
>
> Joe

CITY ISOLATION HOSPITAL

> Tuesday, Jan. 17

My darling Alice: [Typewritten]

I received the boxes today. The candy is delicious. I've been eating it all day. It should help me gain a little weight again. And the bridge game is just what I need to pass time. But it was more enjoyable when we played it together not so long ago. Thanks again, darling.

Did I score today—three letters from you. That is the best medicine that I've ever had.

We got in a new scarlet case. This City Hospital unit is only for isolation, and 40 to 50 beds are cared for at present, primarily by WPA nurses, and they are very efficient. The superintendent is very nice, and as long as she writes my letters, you will receive them.

Pardon the short letters. I'll write a book when I get out of here but just remember darling, I love you.

> Joe

CITY ISOLATION HOSPITAL

Wednesday, Jan. 18

My adorable Alice: [Typewritten]

The bridge game is a life saver, dear. I spend much time playing it, but I warn you that I am not good enough at bridge yet to be your partner.

I am anxious for Dr. Barker's report this week on your health. Of course it will be more favorable than last time. Yes, I'm still well and have 12 days left here.

I believe we can get Louis to come to the wedding this summer if harvest doesn't interfere. Adela and Dennis, of course, will go. I am afraid A. C.'s internship will interfere. More about that later.

Darling, I wish time would fly by, not only the next few days, but rather, the next few months.

I love you,

Joe

CITY ISOLATION HOSPITAL

Saturday, Jan. 21

My adorable Alice: [Typewritten]

I have been up all day and do not even feel tired. And I practically have a new layer of epithelium all over by now. Honestly, I'll be a new man. Now that I can sit at the table, I'll become very accomplished at the card game of solitaire.

My eyes are much stronger now. I'm still on a soft liquid diet. Oh for some gumbo, crab meat, hot tamales, or the other delicious Southern dishes that made me gain weight so rapidly. And, of course, I especially liked the fish.

Right now, like always, I wish I could be 900 miles south with you. Until then, and always I love you.

Joe

CITY ISOLATION HOSPITAL

Thursday, Jan. 26

My dearest Alice: [Typewritten]

It's about time for Baby Snooks and Co. and of course, Bing's program. I hope he sings "Deep in a Dream."

I'm still passing the days trying to digest the bridge plays. They are so interesting that I forget about time, radio, and hospital.

My ROTC enlistment does not make active duty mandatory. It does enable me to get a higher commission in case I enlist in the army medical corps in a time of conflict, which is remote here in U.S.A.

All of our snow is gone by now and it got up to 34 degrees today.

I wish I had your ambition to study, but my alibi is that no books are allowed on contagion. I'll have to catch up when I get back.

Dearest, my thoughts are with you always.

Goodnight, Sweetheart,

Joe

CITY ISOLATION HOSPITAL

Friday, Jan. 27

My Darling: [Typewritten]

Surprise—I've got two roommates, one senior from the Uni. and the other no one else but Dr. David Drummond. I still cannot believe it. Apparently there is some carrier at the Uni. It's grand to see friends from there, but I hate to see them ill.

Dr. Kirk was over. I'll go home for 3–4 days next Monday. Just 4 more days and I'll be out. I'd rather go south than back to work. Darling, I miss you more every day.

All my love,

Joe

My darling—

I just got my first copy of the La. Medical Journal. It is quite inter-esting to read articles by my old profs. There is an interesting article in there about the chronicity of pulmonary tuberculosis. It says that if the patient is kept under treatment until the lesion is radiologi-cally cured, the reoccurrence is less than 1%. That is the best news I've had in that line. Now all I have to do is stick to bed, I guess.

When Dr. Jones came in this evening we had a celebration—an oyster stew celebration. However, my chief cause for celebrating was the thought that by tomorrow or Monday, your isolation period should be over. I surely hope you enjoy a good rest at home.

It's been cold today but is warmer and raining tonight. It is funny how much longer a rainy day seems even though it is spent in bed.

Mother and I had a round of Chinese checkers. I won every game (I have to brag when I get a chance to). That tickled me since she used to not let me win a game an evening.

I hope they forward your letters to you for I don't know whether you are still at Douglas St. or not. If at home, do give my love to all your folks.

Darling, I love you so very, very much. Time would be intermi-nable and the bed hard as rocks if I didn't have my thoughts of you to make the days seem easier.

All my love for my beloved sweetheart—

Alice

ALEXANDRIA
Sun. night, Jan. 29

My dearest one—

Today has been a grand one. Dad came down from his sickbed this morning and started talking about you. He had so many nice things to say, and he is most anxious for more fishing trips with you. He knows you're a fine man in every way because he could tell on the fishing trip.

I hadn't known it before, but it seems that he judges character by the way people act on such trips. Maybe I shouldn't be telling you all this but gee, it makes me so happy.

There's nothing that gives me more pleasure in your absence than Dad winking at me and saying that he's going to write you and tell you that there is no use in your coming back, that Dad has changed his mind about you—and Mother, after worrying audibly about you and wondering if you're getting good food at the hospital, wrinkling her nose and saying, "But I don't like him anyway!" They love to tease and I enjoy them doing it, for I know that they wouldn't unless they cared for you and approved of you thoroughly.

Now darling, I must close. I'm about to use up all of this box of stationery too—but never forget that I love you with all my heart and long for you always.

Love,
Alice

CLARKSON
Monday, Jan. 30

My own sweetheart:

I've waited for this moment for three long, terribly long weeks. I've dreamt about it, just to be able to write to you again. Oh my darling, it will take pages to say all of the things that I want. Oh my dearest, I love you, I love you. If I could only tell it to you in person and once more see that smile on your face, that gleam in your beautiful eyes. Gee, I wish I could sit by your bed again. I'd like to fix your pillows, bring up your tray—and then just sit and watch you. I couldn't ask for anything more. In the past few weeks, I have lived & relived that much too short time between Christmas & New Year's, those precious moments with your hand clasped in mine, that added smile and twinkle in your eyes when the strains of "My Reverie" or "Deep in a Dream" came over the radio. And every moment that I spend away from you makes me all the more anxious to be with you and never leave.

Darling, I can't quite describe how wonderful it is to have someone like you to live for—so lovely and adorable, such a pleasing personality, one who has received so many coveted honors during her college career. Oh, my dear, I'm trying to say that you excel in every way possible. And I could kick myself for getting sick and losing out on our orthopedic training. But, I'll still review the cases when I get back.

Was dismissed this a.m.—and I hated to leave poor miserable Drummond behind. Went to see Dr. Bean and he said, "Go home & don't come back until you feel like it." Well, well—but since I like Radiology & Dermatology, I'll only stay a week. Father & Mother came for me. It was good to see them again.

Now darling, a long goodnight kiss, fix your pillows, put blankets on the bed, turn out the fire, raise the window—and I'll say "Goodnight, sweetheart" and quietly close the door to your room like I did five weeks ago.

I love you, sweetheart,

Joe

CLARKSON
Tuesday afternoon, Jan. 31

My dearest sweetheart:

Now more than ever I admire you for staying in bed so patiently all of this time. After my short illness, I realize more than ever how difficult it is, and it is because of your superb strength of character and determination that you take it with such courage.

I finally got a chance to tell my parents all about the grand time I had at your home this Christmas. Yes, everything in detail—how lovely and sweet you looked, about all the presents, the delicious meals, the fishing trip—everything was so nice.

By the way, darling, we have to give a wedding dance whenever we come to Clarkson. It is customary here—and, my dear, I'll be so very proud to have my friends & relatives meet you. It's music to my ears to have everyone tell me how lucky I am to have you. And how well I know how fortunate I am.

We are listening to some Bohemian music. I get a thrill out of it—and I hope you learn to like it enough to hear it with me sometime. And perhaps we will waltz to it.

Darling, I know my letters the past 3 weeks were very short but, dear, I promise longer ones now. I feel much stronger—although I'm still taking an afternoon nap.

Darling, I wish I could hold you in my arms once again. I love you, darling—can you hear me? I'm madly in love with you—and I will always stay that way. You are my ideal in every way.

Goodnight, sweetheart,
Joe

My dearest Joe—

My eye was just caught by a brilliant green light from my diamond. Now it is blue and now silvery white. Darling, I spend much time just looking at it. However, the symbol—your eternal love—is the dearest possible thing to me.

I'm so anxious to hear from you since you've gone home. Will you get to see Dennis?

I stayed out on the porch for over 2 hours today and enjoyed it so much. I imagine our weather is quite different from yours, especially since yesterday.

Dad is looking much better but says he doesn't feel up to par yet. He has the year's sick leave and is to be retired this fall, and I think staying away more than he would otherwise. But I surely am glad he is. It isn't like Dad to give in, and he must be still feeling pretty "no account," as he says. He maintains he is going back to work tomorrow, but it depends on how he feels. He is going to N.O. next week for a Masonic convention or something and has promised Ray to see a cardiac specialist while there.

I'll bet the days are seeming shorter to you now and I am so glad. Be careful for a while yet though. Goodnight now, dearest, and sweetest of dreams to you.

Love,
Alice

CLARKSON
Thu night, Feb. 2

My darling sweetheart:

I was so glad to receive your letter again. I think they forwarded the others to the Uni. so I'll get them there next Mon. a.m.

I am enclosing the poem you sent. I could not take the one that you sent out of the hospital so I did my best to memorize it. I hope I did not miss too many of the words. It is quite a clever poem.

It almost broke my heart to have to tear up all of the lovely letters that I received from you while at the City. I treasure every word you say so I read and re-read them until I almost learned them too.

Has your father seen the most recent X-ray? I hope that the late hours that we kept during my visit there did not cause you to retard healing. But dear, it was so hard to say good-night. Even a few hours away from you seems like eternity.

Darling, my thoughts were with you constantly. The way you talk, smile, laugh—oh—everything that you do, my dear, is so precious to me.

About the engagement announcement—you could announce it in Alex sooner. And in N.O. probably about the time you get back to work but I think we had better wait until after April in Omaha. Darling, I too want to shout it to the world. I am the luckiest man in the universe.

Goodnight, sweetheart,

Joe

ALEXANDRIA
Thurs. Nite, Feb. 2

My darling—

You can't imagine my joy at receiving your letter. I was thrilled to
see it written in your own dear familiar hand. Now don't think me
unappreciative of the letters written while you were in isolation. I
don't see how you did so well and I was so thankful. But they certainly don't compare with a letter written truly by you.

I am glad you arrived home safely. And do stay until you feel
fully yourself again. You must have been very sick, and you have a
hard five months ahead of you. My, for Dr. Bean to send you home
must mean that they are quite worried about you.

All my love for my sweetheart,
Alice

P.S. I sent last night's letter to Omaha! I can't seem to keep up with
you.

CLARKSON
Sat. night, Feb. 11

My adorable sweetheart:

I am ready to wring someone's neck at the Uni.—my letters are not
coming. They probably think it is a good joke—but I cannot get well
without them. I'll wait until tomorrow's train and then I'll call the
hospital & get them.

It got much, much warmer today—and the thermometer is
settled on the more comfortable side of zero. I hope you are having
warm weather so that you can enjoy your afternoons on the porch.

Is your father back at work already? I'll bet his patients will
be glad to see him back. Why, when I made rounds with him, it

seemed that everyone's face beamed when he came around. I hope my patients like me at least half that much. He taught me a lot of TB & cardiology during that short time—in addition to how to catch four fish on one dead minnow.

How is your mother? We speak of her so often, too—her cheerful manner and pleasant disposition.

Darling, these days without you will soon be over. Until then my memories of you must suffice. I adore you—my own.

> Goodnight, sweetheart,
>
> Joe

ALEXANDRIA
Tues. Nite
St. Valentine's Day

My dearest sweetheart—

Oh, you darling, you'll never know how I enjoyed that phone call tonight. I kept looking forward to it every hour all day. And then, as usual when I talk to you, I almost went speechless, but oh, it was grand to hear your voice. It sounded so very sweet to my ears.

We had quite a fine Valentine's day. The morning mail brought me a pretty box containing a pretty golden sachet on which a little angel sits, all of which is on a red and lacy heart. Painted on the box was To: Dr. Alice Baker, From: An Old Sweetheart (in Mother's printing). It is a yearly joke of ours. Later one friend brought a lovely bouquet of spring flowers, with baby breath, tiny snapdragons, jonquils, narcissi, japonicas, and everything. This afternoon we received some beautiful red carnations, and a western Union boy brought greetings from Dot and Frances. Gee, everyone is too good, but you, darling, are the dearest and sweetest Valentine I shall ever have.

Dot writes of a junior medico-ed who is in the hospital with an extensive pleural effusion, probably tubercular in origin. I'm beginning to believe that we women doctors aren't good investments.

By the way, I didn't get a letter from you today. But I'm sorry you've missed so many of mine. I've written every day. Darling, I love you truly and for always.

Alice

OMAHA
Thu. Night, Feb. 16

My dearest sweetheart:

Gosh, it seems odd to be back—and I had quite a time getting back. It snowed 8 inches in Clarkson, and a little wind made the roads almost impassable, so I took the train to Scribner & the bus from there—arriving here at 3:30.

Had to visit the Dean first & he decided it was OK to start tomorrow morning. The radiology and dermatology services are easy. But the best treat of all on coming back was my letters from you. I had told an intern to "send up my mail" & he thought it meant to take it to my room, so I found 3 wonderful, heavenly letters from you here. Darling, I forgot all about being back and thought just about you.

I am so glad that your father saw the specialist in New Orleans and that he is in good health. I know he will take good care of himself. Darling, I miss you—I love you—that is all I can say, but I mean it with my heart (and also liver & stomach). Now pleasant dreams of you.

Goodnight, sweetheart,
Joe

ALEXANDRIA
Thurs. Nite, Feb. 16

My dearest one—

Good news! My plate taken today shows quite a bit of improvement.

The lesion is about so big **0**—less than half the original size, I'm sure, and Dad got a glimpse of it and said he thought it was resolving as he could see through it better. Dad has already said I can start going to shows, going to visit friends, etc. That darned lesion is so small it seems almost silly to pay any attention to it, but I do get tired pretty easily. That is the only symptom I've ever had, and that is probably just imagination.

And you started to work today—I hope it was fun. Gee, I'll bet it would be a kick to get a call at 2 a.m. again—but I hope you don't have many of them, for a little while anyway.

Mother is just raving about how much weight you lost and how poorly they fed you. I'll bet your mother had a bad time when she saw you—and she certainly must have fed you lots, too. I'm so glad you were able to snap back to normal so soon.

I love you dearly,
Alice

OMAHA

Sunday night, Feb. 19

My darling:

Gosh, we had a rush on emergency films this p.m.—steel in the eye, fractures & chest plates for pneumonia. I abstracted some case records for Deep X-ray & radium therapy. But I would not let that keep me from listening to Charlie McCarthy. I hope that you heard it, too.

I had a grand morning. Stopped in to see Dr. Sucha after church—they live close to the Cathedral. He asked if I wanted to make rounds with him—did I! Gee, it was fun. Went to Nicholas Senn Hospital & St. Joseph's and saw a variety of cases. He is one swell surgeon—and has a wonderful bedside manner. But it did seem funny, me being in a hospital & not wearing white.

Called Dr. Stastny. She has had some cardiac difficulty recently so has been only doing office work for 2 weeks. I must see her soon.

Incidentally, our pathologist Dr. Harold Eggers has spent his life working on cancer and now has developed a "cancerocide" (tetramethyluronium gluconate) which is supposed to destroy by degeneration & liquefaction all of the metastases. It has worked on rats and now they are trying it on inoperable carcinomas to see what it will do on the original lesion as well as metastases. We are all hoping perhaps not this but some related drug may solve the problem someday.

Time is passing so slowly without you near me. I could spend all of my time looking at your pictures—how nice it will be when I can look at you instead. You are so adorable, my dearest—and I am so lucky to have you.

Goodnight, sweetheart,

Joe

ALEXANDRIA
Sun. Nite, Feb. 19

My darling—

How grand to receive such a good long letter with the letterhead of
U. of Neb. on it. It seems like old times again. What sort of work do
you do in radiology? We have no service in that line, but most of
our residents study the X-rays of our patients with us. Do you have
to take all the plates, too?

I have had a most enjoyable time since early Sun. afternoon listening to the programs of Americans All, Immigrants All. The last
two programs have been about the Slavs, Poles and Russians. I've
enjoyed every minute of it, but you can imagine my thrill as they
read the diary of a Czech who settled in Nebraska. Every spring
he said, "This Nebraska is a wonderful country." Every winter he
writes, "This is a frozen wilderness." Ah, but I had no idea of the
number of famous Americans of Slavic descent. And Anton Dvorak
wrote his lovely "New World Symphony" in Prague after a visit to
America. And Chicago has the greatest population of Czechs of any
city excepting Prague. Oh, but the most thrilling part of the program was the emphasis of their love for America and pride in their
new country. All these patriotic talks, programs, pictures, stories,
articles, etc., are certainly making me feel patriotic—but not ready
to fight.

I do so hope July may see us together and that we may always be
together in everything in every sense of the word.

I love you,
Alice

ALEXANDRIA
Monday Nite, Feb. 20

My beloved—

Guess what! I'm getting to be almost a big girl now. I slept in my own room upstairs last night, and it seemed so different. Tonight I get to take my first tub bath. Gee, who ever would think I'd prefer a bath to a movie, but that was my choice today—Ha. See, I'm trying very hard to take care of myself. I just must get back to work by April. I'm anxious to get enough interning in so that I won't have to repeat the year. I hardly believe they will make me do that. But I do hope that when I go back they will let me have OB and Gyn. I was scheduled to have those in Jan. and Feb.

I've been reading your thesis over again. And again I just truly wonder at your brilliance. Honestly dear, it shows many, many hours of hard work, but even more it shows intelligent correlations, new research, and conclusions. I'm enjoying it so much.

Darling, I love you and miss you so darned much. Now, my love, it is time for dreamland and you.

> All of my love,
> Alice

OMAHA
Thursday night, Feb. 23

My darling:

How grand to receive two letters from you today. I am sorry that I didn't get to hear the program "Americans All" that you mention. And, above all, how much you like the Czechs—yes, enough to change to a Bohemian name. Did I tell you what my name means? Little dove. I know we will be as happy as two little loving doves.

I am on the job again—but Radiology is really easy & we spend a lot of time just sitting & discussing the films. Dermatology is easy. I feel a little weak but that is expected—and I rest more than I work.

Ping-pong is the game up in the quarters now—and the competition is keen.

Darling, time indeed is passing slowly—but soon we will be together.

Goodnight, sweetheart,

Joe

ALEXANDRIA

Mon. Nite, Feb. 27

My beloved—

Surprise! Good news!! Dad came home today after talking with Dr. Barker at Baptist Hospital. They both agreed that I had nothing wrong with me deserving attention, and after gradually increasing my exercise I may soon go back to work. Dr. Barker thinks it may be a fungus infection and he cultured a fungus from my sputum, which he injected into a rabbit over 2 weeks ago. The rabbit is still alive and happy. Dad says he just doesn't know what it was. It is still circumscribed and not acting very typical of TB. So he says if it is, there's no need to worry that it will calcify. Needless to say, we had a celebration tonight. I ate with the family, dressed up in your fraternity pin (and my old skirt & sweater), and went to see the Tysons. John Charles was in his night apparel with his hair in curls and the pinkest cheeks. He seems to be about the size of Dennis, according to these new pictures you sent.

Oh, how I longed to have you here for my debut. On return—T° 98.4, pulse 104 (nothing unusual for me). I felt a little tired but no more than could be expected after these months of inactivity. I'm anxious to see the next plate—2 weeks to wait. I hope it will show I may go back to work. Gee, I feel so much better and everything looks 100% brighter.

I'm a selfish pig—writing only of myself. I want you to know how I enjoy the pictures. Dennis is surely a dear, and I was so glad to see your folks' pictures. It looks as if the weather might have been a little cool!

Do you realize that April will soon be here? Oh, what that month means! And then it won't be long until July. Darling, I feel like thanking Dr. Jones every time I see him for interesting me in the possibility of that summer in Mayo's. Such happiness as has been mine since then has never been known. And now, my dearest one—all my love.

Alice

Omaha
Tuesday evening, Feb. 28

My darling sweetheart:

Just finished making rounds with Dr. Cedarblade whose Medicine service I am taking over tomorrow. Have a diabetic patient to do urines & gastrics—I hope he can stay 2 months. I wish I had more time on X-ray. Today I got to fluoroscope a barium & contrast enema. More fun.

The blanket of snow of last night turned out to be about 6 inches here and 12 to 16 inches elsewhere in Nebraska. And did it drift—golly, it surely was fun to see the drifts around the hospital. But it is melting now & the roads are open.

I'll bet you had a grand time with Dot last weekend. Give her my regards, please. But make sure that she does not overwork.

Yes, I am all recovered. In fact, I have started even to play pranks & jokes, which is a sure sign of recovery. And my nickname isn't "shadow" anymore because I have gained my weight back.

I'll be with you in dreamland soon.

> Goodnight, Sweetheart,
>
> Joe

Omaha

Wed. evening, March 1

My adorable sweetheart:

Started off my medical service with a death this a.m. A subacute nephritis who has been on the way out for some time. Have not counted all of my patients yet.

I really got some of the inside dope on this tetramethyluronium gluconate. I have a bronchogenic carcinoma with metastases on which Dr. Eggers started treatment today. I gave 12 units insulin 1 hour before to deplete blood sugar & then about 50 cc of the material. It is a clear yellow liquid—& he has microscopic evidence where it causes a degeneration of the malignant cell because of its unique glucose metabolism. But it is dangerous—and the patient is well aware of it. In this case, the massive necrosis of the tumor mass may cause intrathoracic hemorrhage. I hope not.

Got in a rheumatic fever & a premenstrual syndrome on the woman's side. We have half of male & half of female medicine service.

Drummond's fiancée was here to see him tonight. Gosh, aren't they lucky to be able to see each other everyday—but it won't be long and we will be together. Darling, I am living for that time. I love you so dearly, my own sweetheart.

> Joe

ALEXANDRIA

ALEXANDRIA

Thurs. Nite, March 2

My dearest one—

I was expecting a scorcher of a letter from Dot but it was almost encouraging. Dr. Irwin says it will take 2–3 years before the lesion disappears but agrees that I may go around some if I take it gradually. It is awful to have more than one doctor to tell you what to do, especially when you have faith in both, but darling, I know my Dad will take the best of care of me, and I'll take his word any old time.

Darling, I do so want to believe I'll be OK soon. How could I stand it if it would be 2–3 years before we could be married! But you positively should not be burdened with a gal not up to snuff and—oh, I believe I'll be OK. I feel so darned good now. My dearest, remember me always to the Suchas. I'm so proud of their friendship—but proudest of my own sweetheart.

Love,
Alice

ALEXANDRIA

Sat. Afternoon, March 4

My dearest—

Had another letter from Dot today. Goodness knows I care for her a lot and she has been goodness itself to me, but if she doesn't stop telling me so many cheerful tidbits—as about various people with TB who have gotten up too soon and had to stay 2 years longer in bed, etc.—I'm going to start dreading her letters. I know I shouldn't complain but gee, if that were all I could think about, I'd soon go nuts and really have something to worry about.

I actually believe I'll go to church tomorrow. It will almost seem strange. I'm still feeling mighty good, and my T° doesn't even go up to 99° now. How I hope I can go back to work in April.

Your experience with the new cancerocide is most interesting (I won't even try to spell it). I'm anxious to know your results. Aren't you lucky to be one to use it during the experimental stage.

I love you,

Alice

ALEXANDRIA

Sun. Nite, March 5

My darling—

The minister promised he would make his sermon short, but he kept us 1½ hours. I was glad he hadn't planned a long sermon for I was a little tired before it was over. It was the first time I had seen so many people, therefore I had to dress carefully—so, ahem, no wonder I was tired.

You should see how pretty all the girls look in their new spring outfits—short sleeves, straw hats, etc.—or maybe it's a good thing you can't see them. I'm dying to get up enough to go shopping. Since white was my official uniform for this year, I have the excuse of no new clothes (comparatively) last year.

Darling, I miss you so darned much—but time is passing, if slowly, and it won't be long, I hope, until our dreams come true.

Love,

Alice

ALEXANDRIA
Fri. Nite, March 10

My dearest sweetheart—

You should be with me now. I am waiting out on the sleeping porch and the air is full of the songs of birds. It is warm and breezy—just right. Our sweet olive shrubs have a delightful odor. Now is the prettiest time of our year. I wish so much I could share it with you.

I have a new coiffure (such a fancy name for something so ordinary) tonight, after spending 2 hours at the beauty shop. Then I walked about 4 blocks and with it all, had not one tenth degree of fever. I'm so glad.

You haven't complained of not having enough work lately—I hope it isn't too hard yet.

For lack of anything else, I am reading "The Last of the Mohicans." To my surprise it is interesting. I never stuck to it long enough to find out before.

We're going out to the Base for a free movie tonight—"The Arkansas Traveler." That will be my first night out. How I wish you were here. Then it would truly be a night of celebration.

Oh, darling, I'm happy because of our love—

Alice

OMAHA

Tuesday night, March 14

My darling sweetheart:

I am a little early in writing tonight & will retire extra early—
because, dearest, I've got the first symptoms of "la grippe." But I am
sure it will not last long because I have taken the cold tablets that
your father recommends. And am I forcing fluids. I wish I had some
Bohemian "kminka"—a drink with the smoothness of champagne,
the fragrance of wine and the punch of 15-year bourbon. It is a
good diaphoretic.

Had another dizzy talk with Dr. Poynter. He gave the Nazi salute
in the hall & asked what I think of Hitler's actions today. He doesn't
like him any more than I do.

Gosh, after hearing all of the news bulletins tonight—well, I
wonder how long Hitler will continue in power. Somebody must
stop him. The republic for which my forefathers fought & died—
how they hated the German yoke they had for centuries, and now
it is back—not comparatively benign Hapsburg rule, but malignant
Hitler's. Yes, it makes my blood boil.

Darling, I miss you more & more each day.

Goodnight, Sweetheart,

Joe

Thursday night, March 16

My adorable sweetheart:

The newspaper headlines yesterday made me lose all of the restraint I ever had about uttering criticisms at Hitler. "Czechoslovakia a memory." Maybe it will be a memory to the historians, but not to the Czech people. To them it will always be alive. The century-old hatred is again aroused—magnified a hundredfold. I like the way that they greeted Hitler with "boos."

I shouldn't bore you with my feelings about the new European crisis, but, gosh, that mad man is getting more power every day.

I am so thankful that you are not running any temperature and do not fatigue so easily. Gosh, you won't let me carry you any more, except once & then you must—over the threshold as my bride.

I'm so proud of you, my darling sweetheart.

Joe

ALEXANDRIA
Thurs. Night, March 16

My darling—

And now there is no Czechoslovakia. Oh, that man Hitler—what is he going to want next? Whatever it is, I suppose everyone will rush to give it to him. I still can hardly blame anyone for wanting peace—goodness knows we all want it—but it can't go on like this. It is a new kind of campaigning. Campaigning without war—

I had more fun today. Guess why. I drove the car. Do you realize it is the first time I have driven since I drove Noma? Gee, what memories it brought back to feel my hands on the steering wheel. Happy can't step out to equal Noma—in fact, I'm confident Noma

can't be surpassed, but I got him up to 60 miles per hour just to see
if he still had it in him. He did—but with that Mother got jittery, so
we calmed Happy down.

Oh, dearest, I'm so proud and happy just to think of July.

I do love you dearly,
Alice

ALEXANDRIA
Fri. Nite, March 17

My dearest one—

We should celebrate! The new X-ray shows slight decrease in size
of lesion. I went to talk to Dr. Barker about it this morning. He still
doesn't think it is TB, and I'm to get more sputum for another injec-
tion into the rabbit. Also, he wants me to take the growth to N.O.
and have the fungus identified.

But best of all he says he sees no reason why I shouldn't go back
to work if I watch my diet, rest, etc. So it truly won't be long now.
Gee, to say I'm glad doesn't half express it. I'm finally getting tired of
laziness. This being a lady doesn't seem to agree with me.

Your kminka certainly does sound superb. And I do believe I've
never heard you wax so poetic about anything else. Now you'll have
to promise me a drink of it, but I guess it had better be only a small
one. I seem to remember getting the giggles over 1 1/2 bottles of
beer. Oh, but that was a happy time for me.

Gee, it seems we are missing so much by being so far apart. But
things can't run too smoothly—they wouldn't be half so interesting—and what we have is certainly worth writing and working for.
Did I ever tell you that I love you?

Mother is wondering exactly what and when about things this
summer, but I've told her we can't know exactly until we find out

about Mayo's. She's anxious to start planning things. I'm almost afraid to think of it for fear that no one can have such joy and something might happen. But so long as we can be together, what can happen to hurt us?

> I love you,
> Alice

ALEXANDRIA
Sat. Nite, March 18

My beloved—

I'm just feeling better and better if such is possible. Dad is writing to Dr. Bel that with his permission, I start back April 1. I'm wondering if they will let me start again unqualifiedly. I hope so. I'm sure I can do the work.

We went shopping today, and wonder of wonders, I wore Mother out this time. She always could hold out better than I before. She has a little cold. And Dad isn't feeling up to snuff either. He told me on the Q.T. that he had had an X-ray made and his heart is increasing in size, and his chest still shows slight involvement residual of the flu, he thinks. He is trying to take good care of himself but can't resist fishing trips. And I truly believe that since he enjoys them so much, that it would do him more harm to be deprived of them than not.

Dad and Dr. Jones are going on a fishing trip tomorrow. They will have roasted pig when they get there. When we heard that, Mother and I resolved that we shouldn't be gotten the better of that way, so we'll find something to do tomorrow.

> All my love,
> Alice

ALEXANDRIA
Sun. Nite, March 19

My beloved—

We just got back from visiting the Tysons. I missed seeing John Charles, as that young gentleman had retired. They have a new Chinese Checkers board so you can guess what we did. Mother likes the game so much she plays all by herself.

My, Rumania in the clutches of Hitler—and according to the news flash, she is going to give in. If she does, I guess Hitler's affairs will be much more favorable to him.

Oh, my darling, let us pray we are not drawn into another wholesale massacre!

We had a nice Sunday. Our minister preached such an interesting and valuable sermon on the uselessness and harm of worry, and that worry showed little faith in our Lord.

Darling, I do believe I have a little faith, and it seems to tell me all will be well for us.

I hope I am not being too selfish in praying for that. For my love, how can I even think now of being separated from you after finding that you are my perfect sweetheart?

All my love,
Alice

OMAHA

Tue. a.m., March 21

My darling:

Last night was the first time that I didn't write to you but I do hope that this letter gets there on time.

I was pleasantly surprised yesterday afternoon when my father called & said that he was in town. So I went out to dinner & spent the evening with him.

About 8 p.m. last night I noticed a hang-nail on my left index finger, but it did not hurt. About 9 p.m. the area got tender—so I came home & went to my old room in Ward D with hot packs & neo-prontosil.

It is much better this a.m. It has localized & has not even developed into an inflammation And I feel fine. No T° or white blood count. So please don't worry, darling, I am not taking any chances of getting another infection. Honestly, I am OK and should be out tomorrow. However, I won't go until I have to because I want a little rest—it's the laziness appearing again.

Now, sweetheart, please promise me you won't worry, & I'll tell you how I am tonight again.

I love you, darling, with all of my heart.

Joe

OMAHA

Tues. evening, March 21

My dearest sweetheart:

I'm still in my room on Ward D. Dr. Kirk is my staff man again. I'm feeling grand. There is a little abscess on the lateral surface of my left index finger. Will lance it & have some X-ray treatment tomorrow & gosh, I'll have to go to work soon. Still no T°.

This room hasn't changed much since I was here last—a couple new cracks in the ceiling. Got Cedarblade's radio, so time passes quite fast.

The hospital is having a heck of a time—¼ of the interns are ill. Ross is taking my work again—gosh, I'll owe him about 2 months work soon. One of my cases died—a Hodgkin's who had been seriously ill for weeks.

I'll bet Dr. Poynter will get a hemorrhage when he hears that I am in bed again.

Dr. Schmela was just in. I'll get 50 rads twice a day tomorrow. Comparing it with last time—this is such a smaller infection—that should cure it right away.

I am so glad that your father will retire soon so that he can take better care of his health. Let's hope that the work this spring & summer won't be too hard. Gosh, I am getting anxious for those fishing trips.

Joe

ALEXANDRIA

Thurs. Night, March 23

My dearest one—

Darling, I am so glad that you went to bed at once and I'm really quite proud of you. I'm sure that your prompt attention has aborted it quickly and do take good care of it.

Mother and I stepped out this a.m. to a coffee and this afternoon walked over to see the Tysons. We were lucky enough to get there at John Charles' bath and supper time—and did he show off! He was dancing, standing on his head, and talking continuously. His golden curls are getting quite long and with his pink cheeks, he does look quite girlish. I can't blame Dr. Tyson for wanting them cut. In fact, Bea has about given in. So after they have his picture taken tomorrow for his grandparents (and themselves), they will probably come off.

I wish you could be enjoying days such as we have had today. It has been lovely and warm—almost a summer's day.

Darling, do take care of yourself and rest as much as you can. I know you will, but I must get my word in too. And don't dare forget—

I love you,

Alice

Omaha

Thursday evening, March 23

My sweetest one:

I am having quite a time writing a history on one of my new patients. Ross & I have a system. He takes the present illness & brings the notes up here & I write it up. This is not to be recommended, but it works in this pinch.

I got to stay another day—now hot packs only every 3 hours. There is some muscle soreness in the arm but otherwise I feel swell. Dr. Kirk said I could leave tomorrow a.m. Really, darling, it was nothing to worry about. I got a few days rest.

A.C. is awfully busy with his thesis now. Gosh, just a few more weeks & he will graduate. And then we will probably be separated for a long time. For 16 years we have never been apart over 2 months at a time.

Dr. Kirk is going to N.O. next Saturday for the American College of Physicians meeting. Several other men from the staff are going, too. I told him to call Charity for you about April 1st if you will be there. If not, you will get to meet them here this summer.

Ross just came in with another physical—about 2 lines, and I'm supposed to make 2 pages out of it.

The isolation nursery is 1 floor above, and I can hear the babies all night.

My folks are feeling quite well. Grandmother had the flu but is over it now. I am afraid that I won't get home for Easter this year. It will be the first one I have ever missed.

But, darling, what I miss most of all is the contentment & happiness that I find in your arms. And I'll say it again and again—I love you.

Goodnight, sweetheart,

Joe

Omaha

Friday night, March 24

My sweetest one:

I made rounds of my patients—have a few plenty sick ones. I have been up since this afternoon. I really feel alright but I am taking things easily. Hot dog, I did have a rest. Dr. Kirk will see you next week & tell you it was nothing.

By the way, I told him to call you next Wednesday or Thursday & if you desire to show him around the hospital and town, I'm sure you will like him.

Darling, I do hope that you won't be too busy for a while. Maybe it is because I felt bum when I started back to work, so I hope things are easy & patients are few for a while, at least until you get into the swing of things. And, please, darling, promise me that you will get adequate rest & relaxation, and fresh air. Please do. As for me—I'll sleep every afternoon & take my time about working up patients.

Tonight I can finally get some sleep—it won't be a change of hot packs every hour. That does make it rather inconvenient for the patient, as well as the nurse. So I didn't sleep much. And what's more—my own bed is softer.

Don't worry about me getting any more infections—I'll take all the vitamins, iron, sleep & fresh air available. But best of all, darling, will be the times we can spend together. I do hope we can have a few months vacation before starting work again.

I love you,

Joe

OMAHA
Sunday night, March 26

My adorable one:

Guess what I have been doing this past half hour—you would never guess. Making a kite. Yes, the spring breezes have got me. It has been 10 years since I ever made one, but, boy, this is a creation. It is colossal and I'm proud of it. Now, will it fly?

There are a couple of diabetics in pediatrics who have been wanting to fly a kite for days, so we will go out on the roof tomorrow & have some fun. They can be purchased 2 for a dime at the stores, but I get more fun out of making them for the kids.

No new patients & practically no staff men. All of them have gone to N.O. (the lucky fellows), leaving Dr. Arthur Dunn in charge of both of my services, and he rarely comes out so I'm doing as I please. I wish Dr. Kirk would be on service again.

You should see all of the bearded fellows in Omaha. Union Pacific employees started growing them for the world premiere of "Union Pacific" here next month, and now many men have them— and they say that sweethearts & wives object. No, darling, I have not joined the club yet. The beard that I had in the hospital and the mustache that lasted a short time were enough. Even my long side-burns got clipped shorter.

I was shocked in church today when I learned that next Sunday is Palm Sunday & Easter 2 weeks off. I didn't realize it was that close— which all means, darling, too, that the long-expected first week of April will be here soon. Don't worry, sweetheart, I'm sure that everything will be alright.

I love you,
Joe

ALEXANDRIA

Mon. Night, March 27

My dearest one—

We just got back from seeing "Honolulu." It was the funniest thing I've seen for a long time. Mother got so tickled I thought she would fall out of the seat, and I enjoyed that almost as much as the show. And I must make a note of this—when I make my third million, I hereby resolve to build a movie theater where I can be comfortable (or rather, my legs). Gee, I'll bet you have that trouble, too.

I had a thrill today, too. A letter from Dr. Wm. Carpenter Mac-Carty, Sr.—and I thought I would never get it open. He was very nice, said he was glad I had applied and that he would do anything he could to help me. But that with so many people wanting the fellowship, I must not be too much disappointed if I am not accepted. Bless his heart. I could have kissed him for writing such a nice letter.

My, but I have a lot to do tomorrow. Shopping, packing, etc. Oh, yes, I 'most forgot to tell you. We went fishing this afternoon. It was swell being outdoors, but I didn't even get one nibble. Of course, I'll admit, I hate to use minnows for bait—and I hate to take fish off the line—so perhaps it was just as well. Dad didn't get any large enough to bring home, so I didn't mind so much.

I love you, dearest,
Alice

NEW ORLEANS
Wed. Night, March 29
New Orleans—Hooray!

My beloved sweetheart—

Before I got in the room this afternoon, I heard that I had a package and when I came in—there were the loveliest beautifullest red roses. You are the sweetest sweetheart any girl could possibly have. How I wish I might feel your arms about me—and I would try to thank you as I would like to.

I rather dreaded coming back, but that is all over now and I'm raring to go. I haven't seen many people yet. Gretchen weighs as much now as I do—but that means a gain of twice as many pounds as I did. I hear she is to be allowed to get up gradually starting May 1. She looks grand.

Oh, and I found two letters from you. Gee, I was glad to get them.

I think it was swell of you to make that kite for your little patients. I'll bet they are crazy about you, and how could they help it?

Gee, I hated to leave the folks. I'm just beginning to realize how worried they were about me. I know you were worried too. I hate to think about causing so much trouble to those I love. But now darling, I hope you won't have to worry about me any more.

I hear that there are some very good talks going on here. I'd like to hear some of them—especially the one that Dr. Albert Casey, pathologist, is giving on fungus infections in the lung. But my main job tomorrow is to see Dr. Bel, Irwin, Hull, etc. They told Dot I could have easy services.

Oh, darling, I'm so darned glad to be back and to feel so much better than ever. Now if we could only be together. Thank goodness it won't be long. Now, goodnight, my sweetheart.

All my love,
Alice

'We can lick the whole world together'

April–June 1939

My darling—

Well, whoopee, and three cheers! The first day is over and I feel grand. My feet have objected to being stood on, but they are quieting down now and I feel swell.

I was in the operating room from 8 a.m. to 2:30 p.m. What I hated about it most was missing dinner, but I made up for it at the drug store across the street.

I got 3 new patients today. One is supposed to be a large pelvic abscess. The history is suggestive, but she has also missed 2 periods so I'm wondering. The last was a very sick patient with a badly infected third-degree laceration. Gave her a transfusion tonight but haven't finished working her up—and I'm 5 urines behind—and I quit at 7 p.m., bathed and am resting. So you can see I'm really taking it easy.

I blew up tonight and I shouldn't have, but Dot keeps telling me how to take care of myself, etc.—and I got tired of it. Gee, I don't take being told what to do very well. But darn it, I think I know how to take care of myself and I don't like to ask favors. If I didn't feel I could hold up my end of it, I wouldn't have come back! Sorry to rave to you, but gee, I feel like I'm with you when I write, and of course I enjoy talking about myself.

But not so much as I enjoy hearing about you. Two letters from you today—a real reward for my first day's work.

Oh, Lanny Ross is singing "Heaven Can Wait." I, too, think it is one of our sweetest songs, and one which might have been written for my benefit.

I love you dearly, sweetheart.

Love,
Alice

OMAHA
Saturday night, April 1

My darling sweetheart:

The Hit Parade—gosh, I hope "Deep Purple" is at the top again. It just has to be.

What a surprise, the entire intern staff is back on duty. Cedarblade came back today. Now we will start getting spring fever—particularly with such nice weather. And kite flying is taking a few of the boys out every afternoon.

Only one month of medical service left—golly, I have not learned too much, except how to work up a patient in no time at all.

Darling, I am so very glad that you are getting easy services—and don't think that you have to do all the work. Oh, if I could only help you out. I am certain that together we would & will get more work done. How anxious I am for that time.

Three cheers, "Deep Purple" is tops—and it makes me more lonely for you. I love you, darling. I can never say that enough.

Sweetheart, I have a little information probably to tip us off on what to expect this week. One of my brother Nu Sigs who took 2 years here & two at Northwestern & interned 2 years in King's County, N.Y., just got accepted in Mayo's medicine. I am hoping and praying that all of the acceptances are not out, but I fear that they are. So we won't expect too much & the disappointments won't be so great. However, I'm certain that everything will turn out the best for us.

I'm so glad you liked the roses. I only wish that I could deliver them in person and tell you how I adore you. Now with a prayer for the fulfillment of our wishes in the next few days.

Goodnight, Sweetheart,
Joe

OMAHA
Sunday night, April 2

My darling sweetheart:

Gosh, I'm tired—and I never saw a day when I did less work in the hospital & still called myself an intern. The explanation—my kites. I never saw the interns cooperate so much & have so much fun all year. The wind currents are rather treacherous around the ventilators on the roof. And what a sensation to see a kite clear up in the sky & then the string tear. I almost had a coronary accident when mine took a nose dive. I made another this p.m. & is it a honey. Why, it even holds the record for height.

You should see the quarters tonight—kites, sticks, paste & string all over the place—and my room is no exception. Very typical of the way I used to make kites 10 years ago. Maybe a few more afternoons outdoors would be better than a nap. I'm up to 160 pounds and my appetite is very good—but I still dream of the delicious food that I had this Christmas.

The show "Woman Doctor" is coming to town this week & I'll be sure to see it. There is only one woman doctor for me—and without her my life is empty. Oh, darling, I'm at it again, but, honest, I just

cannot help telling you how I love you and need you near me all of
the time. Dreams of you beside me will soon be true. Days seem
endlessly long when you are away, darling.

Let's hope & pray for good news this week.

>   I adore you,
>   Joe

>   NEW ORLEANS
>   Mon. Nite, April 3

My dearest—

I went to see Dr. Hull today. I've asked him to oversee me. He
ordered a complete workup—urinalysis, blood count, sedimenta-
tion time, etc. He examined my chest but could find nothing. He
wants to see me tomorrow after the lab work is reported. He told
me though, to go right to bed as soon as I quit working, so here I've
been since 7:30 p.m. and I rested from 3:30–5:00 this afternoon.
Lazy me, the habit is still strong with me. I told my resident that I
was going to bed at 7 o'clock every night and I didn't want any fool-
ishness. He said OK, we would only have a ruptured ectopic every
other night then.

It is almost time for Guy Lombardo—see what an early bird I am
getting to be.

>   Goodnight, my sweetheart,
>   Alice

OMAHA

Mon. evening, April 3

My adorable sweetheart:

I guess I'm not a kite flier by trade—at least, I am a little tired from all of that running yesterday. Gosh, I was glad I was busy this p.m. or my prize kite would be lost too. Ross & Francis Richards took all of the string they could buy, borrow, or steal and started 3 box kites—tied 2 blocks apart on the string. Gee, they looked swell for hours—away, way out—& then the wind stopped & string stretched from the hospital for blocks. They recovered one kite & part of the string. We will have more fun tomorrow.

I was correct about my information about Mayo's. I got my letter today—but let's not get worried. I'll tell you tomorrow of my new plans. I do hope that you got in & am expecting a call tomorrow with your good news.

Joe

OMAHA

Tuesday night, April 4

My adorable one:

Spring vacation starts this Thursday. At least we won't be bothered with students & ward rounds for a few days. Had an intern meeting—the WPA is going to replaster & decorate our rooms. Doggone it, I'll bet it takes the rest of the year.

Did some kite flying again. I commandeered all of the string & on a dare let my kite out the full length. It was just a speck in the sky. Now my wrists hurt from winding in that string. But it was so much fun. Big kids—but we make big kites.

Now for our plans. I have sent out about 20 requests for blanks for straight medicine services to start 1/1/40. I don't know what

317

chances exist. Will see about medicine at Crile's clinic in Cleveland next year. Dr. Dunn has some drag in Chicago but I do not know how much. I have also written a letter to Dr. C.A. Mills (the climatologist at Cincinnati) to see if vacancies exist in his department. Do you have any possibilities? I am anxious to hear how you came out at Mayo's. If we do get appointments now, they will undoubtedly start in fall or Jan. In the meantime we could rest or apply to the Medical Bureau in Chicago for positions. But let us leave the latter go for several days yet. I will keep you informed whenever I hear of anything acceptable, & you do likewise. Let us not worry—I'm sure everything will be OK.

Goodnight, Sweetheart,

Joe

Omaha

Wed. night, April 5

My darling sweetheart:

I had a few charts to fix up this evening—one from Jan 22. It is so much work to do them on the wards & so much better to do them to good radio music in the room.

You should hear the kite stories now. Richards was afraid to let his out farther because it might cause international complications as it sailed over Germany. Ross maintained that the war in China made bullet holes in his kite. Well, not to be outdone—my kite went so high & so far it was scorched by the flames of the sun. That stopped them.

Had a very nice letter from Mother today consoling me & hoping we would not be too disappointed. Well, we do have each other, darling—and perhaps our plans cannot come out perfectly this year but, darling, we must be together. I have not heard from any of the hospitals yet. I think we can always get a position through the medical bureau. Do you still want OB & Gyn or Pedy? I'm plenty crazy about medicine yet. And I'm certain I won't want surgery. I should have more to write tomorrow.

My own sweetheart, how I would like to hold you in my arms again—and I soon will.

I love you,
Joe

NEW ORLEANS
Thurs. Nite, April 6

My darling sweetheart—

So Mayo's doesn't appreciate good physicians when it sees them. Honestly, darling, I can't see how it happened that you didn't get in. I suppose we must feel as Dr. Mac said and realize that we were only 2 out of thousands of applicants, and no doubt they could get many with much more experience than we have had. However, I'll lay odds on it that they live to regret not taking you.

I haven't gotten my official refusal yet but am expecting it at any time. I don't know why they are taking so long to break the news.

I'm anxious to know what your new plans are. I've had it intimated that I might get in here if I try yet, but I surely don't want to be away from you. And without you here to counsel with me, I just give up when it comes to planning ahead. I have always been so very fortunate, so I'm just hoping my guardian angel keeps on taking such good care of me.

I don't know if I could bear being separated from you another year. But if we have to wait, I certainly have more to wait for than anyone else could possibly have, for I love you, my dearest.

Alice

OMAHA

Friday night, April 7

My adorable, sweetest, most loveable, perfect darling:

I love you—I love you and I love you. That does not half express my deep feeling toward you. Sweetheart, the new picture is beautiful—I have never, ever seen anything so perfect, except, of course, you in person. I've shown it to everyone around here—but I just cannot get my eyes away from it. I can feel you near me more than ever now.

Darling, I don't see why we should wait any longer with the engagement announcement. Have you announced it in N.O. or Alex already? Oh, how proud I am of you—& I hope this is the last Easter that we will spend apart.

I love you,

Joe

NEW ORLEANS

Sun. Nite, April 9

Easter

My dearest one—

The Easter music is lovely tonight. And was so lovely at church. I've never heard a better sermon. It has been an impressive Easter for me.

Dearest one, your telegram was so sweet—and it was so thoughtful of you to wire the folks. I talked to Mother tonight and she said to tell you how very much they appreciated it. Especially so, since they are both ill. Yes, the flux. I could hardly understand her. She said Clotile was taking good care of them—that she had come back this afternoon, not even taking Easter off. How thankful I am that she is so good to them. Dad is feeling some better. Mother got sick two days after he did.

You are my whole life now, darling, and life will be just a passing of time until we can be together.

> Goodnight, sweetheart,
> Alice

> New Orleans
> Mon. Nite, April 10

My own darling—

What a day! I received the sweetest letter from the dearest person in the world, and it put me on top of the world—even though I too had just gotten my refusal from Mayo's. Darling, you are spoiling me, but I love it. I'm so glad you liked the picture.

I see no reason either for delaying the announcement. No, I haven't officially announced it in New Orleans or Alexandria, but everyone who knows me knows about it. Really, I'm so glad I got that letter today for it fills my mind to the complete exclusion of that Mayo business.

And now, Guy Lombardo is playing a program dedicated to dreamers—how appropriate—and soon our dreams shall come true.

Darling, if you feel we should wait until we have definite plans for work, it will be alright. Goodness knows, with my life with you to look forward to, time will mean little. Of course, I'd hate like everything to delay it, and I hope we don't have to, but I want you to do as you think best.

I still like OB and Gyn and Ped. but as usual, I could easily be interested in any field in which I might have a chance. The residencies in Omaha sound nice, and I'm sure you could get in.

Darling, I do so hope our plans will work out—and I still have utmost faith that they will. Everything must go right for my beloved.

> I love you,
> Alice

OMAHA

Monday evening, April 10

My loveable, adorable sweetheart:

I had a rather long and busy evening doing blood counts, but I had a radio in the laboratory to keep me company. Perhaps if we would not spend so much time flying kites, our work would be caught up. It did get chilly and cold here tonight. In fact, it is supposed to get down to freezing tonight. Gosh, I thought that it was summer already.

Wednesday the WPA starts working in remodeling the quarters. Gosh, that means that we will have the smell of paint & plaster around here for the remaining 3 months. And, I'm not too enthused about having those workers do it. Probably, or undoubtedly, it will take days to months.

Darling, I think we should write for an application blank to M. Burneice Larson, Director, the Medical Bureau, The Pittsfield Bldg., Chicago. Then we have to fill it out and return it. Some of the fellows have received good appointments through her bureau, & possibly we could get close together then. Of course we must be together—& I too want to have a few months rest. That would be swell, a long honeymoon, but we will be on one grand honeymoon all of our lives. Sweetheart, I love you so much.

Goodnight, my dear,

Joe

NEW ORLEANS
Wed. Nite, April 12

My darling sweetheart—

Oh, now I really feel grand. I've been very anxious and yet half afraid to have an X-ray made, but Dot made one for me and darling, well, to be most conservative, it shows no advancement. In fact, it really looks to me as if it shows a little improvement. I'm not going to bank on that until it is officially reported, but if I can work and it gets no worse—why, I feel as if I haven't a care in the world.

If you remember—and I'm warning you, you'd better say you couldn't forget a word we said, especially at a certain time on a certain Christmas Eve—I don't want to marry anyone when I have TB, much less you, for my love means that I want everything to be the best for you that I can make it.

Oh, no wonder I am so thrilled.

I guess I'll have to delay my talk to Dr. Hull about possible residency applications. I hear he is to be married tomorrow, and I wouldn't be a bit surprised if his mind might not be on something else. What do you think? He gave us a talk tonight on electrocardiography. He and Dr. Richard Ashman, chief of our Physiology Dept., wrote a book on it and I think it is very good—but perhaps I am prejudiced.

Darling, I hope it isn't a shock to you but I've discovered something—I love you with all my heart, and I'm afraid it is a chronic affectation. In fact, I'm sure it will last until—and after—my life, for you are all my life, dearest.

Alice

OMAHA

Thursday night, April 13

My adorable sweetheart:

Wayne King is on the air—it is ages since I heard him, which means that I have not been up this late for a long time. Yes, it's way past my bedtime—11:00. I was down at the Med-Reserve officers meeting tonight. I don't like all this business about war, but the chances are very remote about there being any. And it does give us a different viewpoint.

I have talked with Colonel Hall & he has put me on the list for an army hospital vacancy & can get me into CCC—but we will let that wait.

We are having spring again—but kite flying is neglected because of work. Did I tell you that my kite is white because it was up in the Milky Way—and that it came back with stardust on it the other evening?

Oh, darling, I dream of the time when I'll again hold you in my arms.

Goodnight, Sweetheart,

Joe

NEW ORLEANS

Thurs. Night, April 13

My beloved—

I just wrote The Medical Bureau for an application blank. Honestly I'm afraid I shan't know what line to apply in for I'm in a quandary. I'm beginning to discover how little I know about Gyn—and how blind my fingers are.

Had quite a day today. We had two interesting operative cases. The first was a pelvic mass, believed to be an ovarian cyst, but which decreased surprisingly in size at the recent menstrual period. It turned out to be a soft benign tumor of the uterus. The second was a 13 year old colored girl with the chief complaint of uterine bleeding. She had a large cystic ovary, about the size of a grapefruit, on the left side. On the right of the ovary was a smaller but also cystic ovary, and the ovary was replaced almost wholly by fibrous tissue. However, due to her age, the right ova was left in after one cyst was removed and the others punctured. I'll bet she'll be back soon and that one has to be removed.

We're having field day Saturday—3 laparotomies and a vulvectomy on Tulane service, and 3 laps and a D&C on Independent service. Now the question is, how can I be in both places at once!

Are you interested at all in Public Health? I have always thought it would be a good line—and maybe especially so with the possible advent of gov't controlled medicine.

Darling, even Dot & Dr. Irwin have agreed my lesion is getting smaller. Only 1/3 its original size. So I feel like I could conquer the world now. But what I really want is to be at your side and watch (and help a little if possible) you conquer this old globe. I love you dearly, my darling—

Alice

OMAHA
Monday night, April 17
8:45

My darling one:

Perhaps I should not tell you this and destroy your desire to come up north, but we had snow today. Honest. All day too—and the wind whistled like a good midwinter northerner. Now it has turned to rain. Needless to say, it is nasty outside.

The Medical Bureau should be able to secure us something for 1 year or so if everything else fails. It has a $2 registration fee. I'll write and explain that we wish to be together—or within a few miles if possible. If I could get something through them in La., would you stay at Charity? Probably a locum tenens might be very valuable experience for a few months in order to tide us over until appointments start again. You apply in whatever specialty you desire. We'll also consider Public Health—but, truthfully, I had never thought of it.

I'm certain that everything will be OK for us. We must remember that we have been infinitely lucky—in finding each other, in having our love & seeing each other a few times this year.

So, since we did not get what we wanted, perhaps, darling, it is all for the best & we will eventually be thankful. I know we'll be together soon—and being together, sweetheart, will mean happiness.

I adore you,
Joe

NEW ORLEANS
Mon. Night, April 17

My dearest sweetheart—

Dr. Fader was talking to me again today. He says we could both
have gotten in here if we had applied earlier, and may be able to yet.
I do wish I knew exactly what we should do. I think I shall try to
talk to Dr. Weilbaecher and ask him if there are any vacancies that
might be filled in October. I don't think they are supposed to take
new staff members except in July, but there are usually a few excep-
tions. If not, do you want to apply here anyway?

One of our visiting men, whom I know only by sight, was inquir-
ing about my plans. He asked if I were going to practice or get married. I retorted that I hoped to do both. Then he said, "You two are
certainly letting yourselves in for it. I can't imagine anything worse
than marrying a doctor." Whom do you think he was thinking of,
you or me? After all we're both going to marry a doctor—Ha. He
wouldn't say that if he knew you, for I can't think of anything worse
than not marrying my doctor. He is so wonderful.

Gretchen is getting up for a ride in a wheelchair every day now.
She looks wonderful. She is always asking about you. Let's hope she
will have that pleasure soon. How I love to show off my Joe—for he
is the dearest sweetheart ever.

Love, all of it,
Alice

NEW ORLEANS
Tues. Night, April 18

My beloved sweetheart—

I talked to Dr. Weilbaecher today. He said all the residencies in Medicine and Surgery were filled and several people left over. He said it might be possible for me to get in as a resident in Tulane Pediatrics, if one of the fellows drops out as he seems to be considering. However, he said that someone from away from here would probably have no chance this late since there were still boys from here who wanted residencies and it wouldn't be fair to give them to someone from away from here. He said it was too late to apply, but that he would be on the watch for anything which might come up and would let me know. However, even if we both got in, I'm afraid it would have to be July 1, 1939. The only other opening that might be possible here is on the teaching staff of the pre-clinical courses, as the clinical staffs are made up of residents and on up. So, it looks to me as if our chances here—for next year at least—are rather slim.

You are well known in Omaha, and wouldn't you like to be connected with a teaching institution? If you find what you want in Omaha, don't refuse on my account.

I can imagine how grand it will be when all this business is settled. But heaven for me will be when I am truly yours.

Goodnight, dearest,
Alice

OMAHA
Friday, April 21
1:00 a.m.

My darling one:

I understand about the residencies there—undoubtedly difficult to get in in July & much worse now. But, sweetheart, would it be possible for me to get in with some M.D. there? Undoubtedly very few take assistants, particularly strangers, but I would be willing to work for anyone for a year. Or how about the interns who drop out? I feel certain that I would have a much better chance to get in if I'd be around there—& I know darn well that I can more than satisfy anyone I'd work for.

I'm not boasting, sweetheart, but I've got confidence in myself & you. And we both know that we could have made Mayo's this year if we had not been ill.

I'd like a year in Anatomy, but if you find anything, let me know. The Pedy residency for you sounds good and just what you want.

I expect to hear from the Bureau soon, so let's not do anything definite for a few days yet.

Oh, darling, the time does pass so very slowly—I adore you, darling, and I love you.

Joe

NEW ORLEANS
Sun. Night, April 23

My dearest one—

I have really had a nice day. I worked all morning—2 new patients, a blood transfusion, lab work, etc., but this afternoon Dot and I went with her brother Charles to her home in White Castle. Her dad looks pretty bad, but seems pretty cheerful. He can hardly be understood when he speaks, and both legs are markedly edematous. I feel so sorry for him.

It was a great trip, though. It is still cool and looked rainy all day, but didn't rain much. The river is coming down quite a bit, but the farmers need rain. The airline highway is completed to the N.O. city limits and is surely a grand road. It was lovely driving at twilight. Charles prophesied a long life of happiness for the two of us. I believe—and hope—he is right.

You should have heard Marie, Charles' wife, complimenting my ring. She agrees with me that it is lovely and very tasteful. She says you must have very good taste. Oh, darling, do you know I am so proud of that ring. It is undoubted the loveliest one I've ever seen, and it is so very precious to me.

I have one true and one potential diabetic on my ward—more work! I've never had a service yet on which I haven't had a diabetic. I hope I get to manage these by myself. I'd like to see if I could control them without any suggestions from residents, etc.

I'll try to talk to Dr. Beryl Burns, Chief of Anatomy Dept., tomorrow. I'm beginning to believe you want to come here to N.O.—how about it? The fact that I'll have to go to work July 1 if I take the Pedy. residency had seemed a drawback to me, but I guess I shouldn't mind that so much. I do wish we could find jobs for October through the Bureau. I talked to the folks tonight and they are fine. They are very glad we put our applications into the Med. Bureau. Have you sent your pictures in yet?

Darling, every breath is a prayer that we may find our happiness together. Goodnight, dearest sweetheart—

Alice

NEW ORLEANS
Monday Night, April 24
10:45

My dearest one—

Today has really been a field day. I've been working straight through
all day and have to get up at 1 & 5 a.m. to give antipneumococcic
serum—a 2nd day post-operative case. And I had looked forward to a
nice restful day, since it has been raining and very enticing to sleep.

And darn it, I missed Guy Lombardo. I surely hate to miss him
for I always feel you are listening, too.

I went to see Dr. Burns. I asked him if he ever took any recent
graduates in his dept. He answered that he would if he could but he
wasn't allowed to. He told me to see Dr. D'Aunoy, that they should
find something for me to do—teach the nurses, if nothing else.
Well, I don't think I shall take his advice. I hate like the very devil to
beg—and that's the way I would feel to go to D'Aunoy. I'm allergic to
that man! The very thought of him makes me feel bad the rest of the
day. Oh, I'll calm down with time, and if you find something here it
will be swell. I haven't heard from my Pedy residency yet. I probably
won't get the chance at it.

Yes, darling, it is indeed a challenge for us. And one we will
undoubtedly meet. As long as you don't get the small end of it
because of me, I'll be more than satisfied.

Darling, if we are truly going to be married this summer, can we
start making definite plans? If, however, it depends on our jobs, I
guess we can't still—but dearest, the thought of such happiness is
more than I deserve. You are too sweet, kind, precious & lovable for
any mere human girl—but I do love you deeply.

Alice

NEW ORLEANS
Wed. Night, April 26

My beloved—

Dr. Hull came back today, and you should see the change in him. He's just bubbling over with happiness and has a pat on the back for everyone he sees. He surely is one swell guy, and I am happy for him. He gave us another talk on electrocardiography. It is a strain to keep up with him (I've used my brain for so little this last year—except for thoughts of you, which require no effort), but I believe I've managed to keep up so far.

I got my application for a weekend off today and tried to find out what service I have next—but since I am the problem child, they haven't fixed it up. I'm getting anxious for a month of Surgery now.

One of the nurses gave me the name of 4 hospitals in Houston. I may write to see if they have any openings this year. That should be a nice place to be. But your letter saying you were too willing to let the Med. Bureau take care of things sounds good to me. I believe it is the best way and that we'll be able to find something good.

It is now less than 9 weeks until our internships will be over. Oh, what a happy time I am looking forward to with my beloved.

I love you,
Alice

OMAHA

Friday, April 28

My sweet, lovable, adorable darling:

Things have happened rather rapidly during the past day or two. First, I may have a chance to get into the Maybury Sanitarium in Northville, Mich., 8 mi. from Detroit. It is a large TB institution —$150 per month & maintenance. The advantage is that it is close to Detroit & we could get into Harper's or Henry Ford hospital next year. Also it is 60 miles from Ann Arbor & we could take some work there. If you desire, I am certain you could take the special clinical courses they have to offer. The disadvantages are, of course, obvious, but I frequently wonder if the chances of picking up TB are less in an institution than in a general hospital as we are now. I will not know definitely for about a week. It would give us an "in" with other institutions. Let me know your reaction.

Also, I applied for medicine residency at Presbyterian at Chicago to start Sept. 1st. I also sent my application to Dr. Herbert Schattenberg at Tulane—I do hope it comes through. I let him know that I would like 2 years Path but what I really want is to follow that with 2 years medical work.

Remember, sweetheart, I love you madly and want to be near you always.

Goodnight, Sweetheart,

Joe

NEW ORLEANS
Friday Night, April 28

My dearest one—

I had a scare this morning when I was told I was to be put on ambulance duty. That means 24 hours on duty and 12 hours off. I was afraid it would be pretty hard on me, the way I've been resting all the time, and Dot and Dr. Irwin jumped all over me for even considering doing it. But when I went up to talk to Dr. Bel's secretary, she said they had decided to give me Tulane Surgery instead for one month—and then OB. I went over the new ward with the present intern. He has only 13 patients now and none acutely ill, so it doesn't sound so hard. Gee, I'm surely looking for soft jobs—eh! But I still don't want to take any chances, for more reasons than one.

I'm full of hopes and dreams. I'm sure everything is going to turn out for the best with us. All my love, dearest sweetheart.

Alice

OMAHA
Sunday evening, April 30

My adorable darling:

This has been a wonderful day—I mean really swell—and primarily because of the engagement announcement. I stopped at the corner pharmacy for some coffee after church, and there were about 25 dozen nurses there with the society page. So I practically bought out the drug store—including a box of cigars for the boys here. Oh, sweetheart, was I happy to see your picture—and it is so nice.

And all of the hospital was offering me congratulations, & staff men called me up. I only wish that you could be here.

Such remarks as these: "Gosh, she is good looking." "I knew she was real intelligent but she is good looking, too." "You surely are lucky." "How did you rate such a nice girl?"

Sweetheart, I am so anxious to have you here and meet everyone. And I am so very proud of you.

Tomorrow we get moved out of our rooms & five of us will sleep on the porch. And, worst of all—Drummond is one of them & I had enough of his snoring at the pest house—the city isolation hospital.

Am starting on surgical service in the a.m. Have not made ward rounds yet, but I believe we have some good cases.

Talked with Dr. A.D. Cloyd today—my chances at Ford Hospital are pretty good for next year. I am waiting for your letter and also reply on my applications. Have not heard from the Maybury hospital yet.

Oh, sweetheart, I adore you—heart and soul.

Joe

NEW ORLEANS
Tues. Night, May 2

My beloved sweetheart—

I called Dr. Schattenberg today. He said he was very, very sorry but the vacancy had been filled. He asked me to give you his regards. I hear that Dr. Nix takes doctors in his clinic. There may be an opening here. He has a large medical and surgical clinic on St. Charles Avenue and has a wonderful practice. He and Ray were good friends. His name is Dr. J.T. Nix—and couldn't you tell him you could see him personally in July? Gee, that would be swell.

How many months of surgery do you have? Mine has been very easy so far, but tomorrow will be my first Tulane day, and they say that you usually get 2–6 observation room cases. The students write our histories, use our physicals, and do our lab work. It certainly has been nice so far.

Darling, I'm so proud of you—and I do love you so much. I just know everything is going to turn out alright for us. What have you heard from Michigan? It sounds good except as you say—the fact it is TB. Gee, I'm as anxious to hear from you again as if I hadn't heard today.

I love you with all my heart.

Alice

NEW ORLEANS
Wed. Night, May 3

My own darling beloved—

The Ford Hospital offers a wonderful opportunity, doesn't it? If you don't mind the hospital being a tuberculous one, it sounds very good. I personally have always been very interested in TB—and you are probably right that there should be less chance of contracting it in a TB hospital where excellent precautions are always taken.

I've been thinking seriously of trying to get a job teaching—anatomy, preferably. I have always looked forward to responsibility with dread—goodness knows I didn't show it in choosing my profession—but I would have much more time for home (which, with you, will always be the foremost thing in my life) and without so many depressing worries. Besides, I believe I would like it and I might be able to make a go of it.

Paul Whitman's song of the week—"Our Love"! How very appropriate. I truly do feel our love everywhere, and it is a constant joy to me. How empty was my life before I met you.

Alice

NEW ORLEANS
Fri. Night, May 5

My own dearest one—

I was so thrilled tonight. To hear your voice is wonderful—oh, darling, you are the dearest person on earth.

I had a feeling all week that Friday was going to bring us good news. Don't ask me how I knew it—I just felt it in my bones. And this morning as I was coming down the elevator I saw Dr. Hull waiting on the first floor. He motioned to me and said he had received a letter from the Medical Bureau. Then he asked me what I wanted to do next year. So I answered that I wanted to get married and I wanted to find work near you. He asked me what you wanted to do and when I answered Internal Medicine, he told me that Dr. D'Aunoy had told him he could have three fellowships in medicine and that he had two already and that if Dr. D'Aunoy would let him, he would hire both of us.

You can imagine what I answered when he asked if you were a good man. I was so proud to be able to brag on you.

He said he wanted young men who had just finished their internship, whom he could train himself. So I left with all sorts of hope in my heart.

This afternoon he asked me to come to his office and he took your name, address, etc., and said he was going to talk to the dean right away and he hoped he could take both of us. And, gee, there was never a longer afternoon. I had a continuous prayer in my heart. And finally when 7:30 came at last, I called Dr. Hull and he said Dr. D'Aunoy agreed he could take both of us. The only thing which isn't settled is the salary. But he said they would give us at least $75 a month each. And darling, as you say, we can live like kings on that.

I tried to get you right away, but the operator soon informed me that you were out. Then I phoned Frances and told her to bring on the beer, we had something to celebrate. And darling, I am on my third bottle, so if you have any trouble reading this letter, just remember New Year's Eve and you will understand why.

I'll ask Dr. Hull when we can have time off for our most momentous step. I believe he is still in seventh heaven over his own marriage, so he will probably be most sympathetic.

I phoned Mother and she is overjoyed. She said it was almost too good to be true—but we'll see that it does come true. Oh, my darling, think what it means—more than we had even dreamed of. When I think of how we can spend our time together, and have an apartment all our own. Oh, darling, it is indeed heavenly.

> Goodnight, dearest sweetheart—
> Alice

OMAHA

Sat. night, May 6

My darling one:

Sweetheart, I still can't believe it—and am so anxious to get your next letter. It is something that we never expected—and so much more than we asked & prayed for.

I am also anxious for their reply to my application.

Oh, darling. Days are just so much torture while we are apart. But the time is getting shorter and shorter. And soon, darling, we will be together.

I live only for you, my adorable one.

> Goodnight, sweetheart,
> Joe

NEW ORLEANS
Sat. Night, May 6

My precious one—

Darling, I am still walking on air.

I didn't get to see Dr. Hull again for I was in the operating room from 10–2:30. Had a laminectomy. I didn't get to see much of the operation. I guess it was because Dr. D.H. Echols hadn't realized I was a doctor. But he surely found out. When it was over he said, "Miss, what are you, a student or a nurse?" I was angry and snapped back, "I'm a doctor." When he found out I was the intern on the case, he only answered, "I didn't know that." But I'll have to hand it to him. He is a pretty operator.

Oh, darling, aren't we fortunate. Goodness, I consider myself about the luckiest person alive. Darling, isn't it grand? It is better than anything I had ever expected—especially getting to live outside the hospital. I do hope it lives up to what we believe it to be. I guess I go to extremes too much, but as far as I can tell, it sounds darned good to me.

Mother was quite thrilled with the announcement. She says she's really beginning to realize now that I'll soon be married. Oh, my dearest one, I am so very, very happy. I do so hope our plans and dreams all work out as lovely as they have so far. I love you—with all my heart, liver, and stomach.

Alice

OMAHA
Sunday night, May 7
8:35

My sweetheart:

I'll be watching the mails very, very closely for that letter from Dr. D'Aunoy—oh, darling, it is so wonderful. That means that we can do most of the things that we expected and yet be together. Picnics, tennis, swimming—and all in Romantic New Orleans. No more 1,103 miles apart. It will be heavenly.

I wish this time would pass more quickly—every minute away from you is a century wasted. Darling, I love you. Every beat of my heart is calling for Alice.

Goodnight, Sweetheart,

Joe

NEW ORLEANS
Sun. Night, May 7

My dearest one—

Mother just called me. She said she was so excited she couldn't sleep Friday night. She and Dad are almost as happy as we are. What do your folks think about it? It has that same old objection, only being too far away from them now. I do hope we shall be able to see them often.

Frances has been trying to persuade me to take the rest of my vacation, and she has about persuaded me, for I would love to be home on Mother's Day—and now we shall have so much to say and so many plans to make.

My goodness, I can't get over how easy my surgical service is. No new patient today and I've had practically the whole day off. I went to church. It was communion service—and to complete it, the scripture was the 13th chapter of Corinthians. It seemed a special opportunity for me, and my heartfelt thanks and gratitude were sincerely given.

I love you,
Alice

NEW ORLEANS
Mon. Night, May 8

My beloved—

I talked to Dr. Hull today. He got your letter and showed me your picture, as if I couldn't remember what you looked like, he said. We are entitled to a month's vacation, but he thought we had better take only 2 weeks so early. He said we had better wait until the last two weeks of July to take our vacation, so we could get started before we left. So, my dearest one, I suppose we can plan on the last two weeks of July for our big plans!

He is very enthused over our work next year. There will be one full-time man—Drs. Robert Bayley, Charles Allen, Robert Chester Lowe, and one who hasn't come yet—on each service, white and colored, male and female. And he is to be in charge of one half and Dr. Julius Bauer, recently of Austria, in charge of the other half. And we all rotate every 3 months, so we get all services and all the professors. He hasn't decided yet how he is to work in contagious and tuberculous services. Gee, doesn't it sound marvelous!

He said the dean had said that he didn't know how it would be to have a married couple working together, but Dr. Hull had assured him that it would be fine—and I echoed that.

At any rate, perhaps we can get settled on a date now. Shall we plan on about July 16–18 or some such? Darling, stop me if this is going too fast, but I'm hard to hold down these days!

I'm planning to go home Sat. and stay through Tues. Frances is still more than willing, so I might as well take advantage of it.

Oh, darling, I am so very, very happy. I'm so anxious to hear from you. Your letters mean so much and now, goodnight, my dearest one.

All my love,
Alice

NEW ORLEANS
Wed. Nite, May 10

My dearest sweetheart—

I went to Dr. Hull's lecture on electrocardiography tonight. He told me that everything is now official. Bless his heart, he surely is sweet to us. I do hope you'll like him as I do—and think him as good a teacher. And you can just tell he enjoys teaching.

You surely have a lot of work to do. I'm lucky—I have students on the ward to write complete histories and do all the lab work, except on observation room cases. I only have two operations scheduled for tomorrow. I'm glad for I have a new patient I haven't yet worked up. The ward is crowded, too. I'll leave either Friday night or Saturday a.m. and come back Tuesday night. I'm lucky to get to be with Mother on Mother's Day.

Oh, darling, the time passes more and more slowly! When will you be able to come down? Can't you leave there a few days early since you are supposed to start in here July first! Oh, darling, I'm so anxious to be with you.

All my love is yours,
Alice

Omaha

10:20 Sat. night, May 13

My darling one:

Had some nice news. Father and Mother are coming up for Mother's Day tomorrow—and I believe I can get off practically all day. Gee, there will be so very much to talk about. All about plans for this summer. I'll bet you will hear ringing in your ears all day.

Honestly, darling, I am crazy about the Fellowship. It is just what I wanted—and, really, my secret desire has been to live in N.O. someday, to be where you spent your life, to meet your friends & be in the same environment. But I feared even to wish & pray for that because I thought that it was asking too much.

Only one thing is holding me back from broadcasting it to all of Omaha. You said Dr. Hull said it was all official. I have not heard from him yet. But I don't want to hurry them. As long as it is cinched, that is all that matters.

Now, instead of waking up at night & having nightmares about what & where we will be next year, I awaken with thoughts of you and dream of our own little apartment in Romantic New Orleans. And my dreams just do not stop.

I am certain that we will learn more medicine together than any other way. We can see each other's cases—like unofficial consultants.

Darling, I am really so very happy that we will get the positions. It is so much better than our applications up north. And I also want to know what the southern clime will do to an overstimulated Yankee.

Sweetheart, I am very interested in cardiology and want to hear & study under Dr. Hull.

I am laying the groundwork to get out of here the 25th of June. I should be in N.O. the 29th. After that we won't have to be separated ever again.

Goodnight, Sweetheart,

Joe

ALEXANDRIA
Sun. Nite, May 14

My beloved—

Oh, my darling, you can never know how happy your call this afternoon made me. It does me so much good to realize you are happy about the whole thing, too—and your voice was so strong and sounded happy, and oh so dear to me. Mother and I just sat and talked about you and gee, we're so happy together. Then we began to realize how much there was to do and how little time to do it in—for I will be on OB the last month and won't be able to have any time off in the daytime. And it will only be 6 weeks until you come and 8 weeks (approximately) until we can be married. Gee, you haven't even said all these wedding plans were agreeable, and here I am planning full speed ahead. Darling, are you sure we can be married at home? For if we can, I want to dress up in a veil, white dress, etc.—and if not, that wouldn't be suitable for a wedding in the chapel. Oh, yes, I think an 8 a.m. wedding would be nicest. It can be informal and yet very nice. Then right after the ceremony, we plan to have a wedding breakfast—just for my best friends and all of yours who come down. I imagine it will be about 35 people. Say, can't A.C. take his vacation that early and come down? If you think it will be OK, I'd like to write and ask him to come, too.

And oh, yes, if you or your mother will send me the list of those to whom you want invitations and those to whom you want announcements sent, we could get started on that too (if I ever get my list made out). Darling, if you don't answer soon—enthused or vice versa—about all these plans, I'm going to be unable to stand it. It's awfully tough to try to plan things without having you near to consult, and I do so want them to be pleasing to you, too. For darling, I love you forever and always—

Love,
Alice

NEW ORLEANS
Tues. Nite, May 16

My dearest one—

Well, I'm back. Frances has really had some work. The ward is crowded and the same diabetic is cutting up again. They amputated her leg today, gave her 780 calories by infusion—and now the job is to get her controlled again. I surely hope it doesn't take long.

I hated to leave home today. It is fun to have no responsibilities and to relax at home. The folks are so very, very glad we are to be here in N.O. Dad says you must have a fishing trip soon.

Darling, will you see about the arrangements for our wedding— I mean, asking the priest, or telling me how to do it, and to see about the pronouncing of the banns, etc. I don't know much about it, but if you'll tell me I'll try to do my part, OK?

Gee, it is going to be fun looking for an apartment, but I surely don't want to do it by myself. Dot says I may stay here with her the first two weeks in July. Then we could lease the apartment for July 1. I do want us to go together to look for them, and I wouldn't have much of a chance to look for one being on OB duty in June.

Darling, the very thought of this summer thrills me and makes me so happy.

> All my love, dearest one,
> Alice

OMAHA

Friday night, May 19

11:00

My darling sweetheart:

Golly, it is hot here. I'll be very well acclimated to hot weather by July. Today seemed like a mid-August day. And it is much too hot to work on the wards—but not for tennis.

I started to do some shopping today—and ended up getting a pair of shoe laces. Perhaps I need you along to help me.

I will write to Father Clement Nuedling at St. Francis Xavier Cathedral and make all of the wedding arrangements. I think the 8 a.m. time should be more acceptable to him. I will let you know as soon as I hear from him.

As for the apartment—perhaps you could have several addresses or prospective vacancies spotted & then we can see them in July. I would prefer a garage nearby. But any place will be heaven with you.

Darling, when I think of the delightful times we have had together, each meeting richer & fuller of thrills, and what a lifetime of happiness we have before us—why, it is the most perfect thing that could happen.

Will the magnolias be in bloom when I come? It should be time for a full moon. We must spend an evening at Pontchartrain Beach.

In all of my rambling, I'm trying to tell you how happy I will be from July on, and how wonderful you are, and the same old story—I love you.

Goodnight, Sweetheart,

Joe

NEW ORLEANS
Sun Night, May 21

My dearest sweetheart—

Dot took me with her to see the new hospital today. Dr. Irwin wanted her to help him, and before her work started we slipped away and did some exploring. My, I hadn't realized how large one floor could be—and there are more blind alleys, stairs, etc. Gee, I had to look out of a window to be able to tell anything about where I am.

But the building is marvelous. So many nice examining rooms in the clinics, several emergency operating rooms, small wards with adjoining nurses' offices, interns' offices, and a nice laboratory between 2 wards. Gee, neither the doctors nor the patients will know how to act after this hospital. I hope they furnish guidebooks to the doctors, anyway.

When you were talking to the priest in Alexandria, did he tell you anything about me having to take some instructions? Dot says that in Archbishop Rummel's jurisdiction, the non-Catholic must take instructions beginning 6 weeks before the marriage. I do hope they don't make me promise a lot of things. I guess I'm stubborn and prejudiced. I'll try to be good.

Darling, above all and everything, I do love you truly.

Alice

OMAHA
Wed. night, May 24
8:30

My darling one:

Well, tomorrow we are operating on two cases the staff man hasn't seen yet again. That happens often. I felt like growling this a.m.— Dr. J.R. Nillson was in a hurry so did the appendix himself in about 15 minutes instead of my taking, well, a lot longer.

The new Charity must be perfect—gee, I am so anxious to get there. But any hospital is tops as long as you are there.

Darling, when I talked to Father Nuedling last December, he stated that as far as he knew you might not have to take the instructions but he would know later. But, honestly, sweetheart, if you do have to take them, please remember that in no way whatsoever are we trying to force anything upon you. The 6 one-hour lessons are only to tell you of the Catholic point of view on certain problems. The priests giving them are very liberal-minded and will answer any questions you would care to ask. It is just to acquaint you with certain of our theories. I am sure that we can work it out well.

Three more days & another week will be gone, and the month will soon be over. The days of June will be unbearably long—but starting the 29th they will be heavenly.

Goodnight, Sweetheart,

Joe

NEW ORLEANS
Sat. Night, May 27

My beloved—

Darling, I'm ashamed of myself to have said anything about the instructions. It was just a surprise to me, but I don't mind—and I shall welcome the opportunity of discussing those problems and yes, I may have some questions to ask. I do hope I shall not interfere with your religious pursuits. If I do, it will certainly be unintentional. I am truly sorry we are not of the same beliefs—but they are essentially the same, dearest, and surely we will be able to work out everything. Maybe as I learn more about Catholicism, I shall accept more.

Darling, it will soon be June and how happy I will be for the 29th. I am looking forward to it so much—the fulfillment of all my dreams.

Love,
Alice

NEW ORLEANS
Tues. Night, May 30

My dearest one—

Hurray! Today is the last Tulane observation day, and as you might guess, I shan't be a bit sorry. It's funny. Even the nurses dread Tulane day. It is funny that everything seems to happen on those days.

I had two observation cases so far. One was a subacute appendix. The surgery resident was thrilled and honored at being allowed to do it under supervision. Imagine, he's been a surgical resident a whole year and is grateful to get to do a simple appendectomy—and you get to do them in your internship. It just goes to show how smart my honey is!

You should have heard me blow up tonight. I really let off steam and I really feel better now. I've been trying to give two infusions since 7 p.m.—and finally got them done after 9 p.m. We've been giving these infusions twice daily for a week but never yet have they had enough glucose—and it never occurs to anyone to send after any until I ask them to get the infusions ready. Gee, we surely need an efficiency expert around here. They have the excuse of the crowded condition, etc., but it won't be any better in the new hospital unless someone gets behind everyone and makes them start using a little common sense.

Which applies to the interns too (myself not excluded). Dr. Bel gave us a raking over the coals today about being behind with the charts. It was the first time he has ever spoken to us, but it wasn't any too pleasant. He read out the names of those with incomplete charts in the record room and the number of charts they were behind. Thank goodness my name wasn't on it, for once. He ended up by saying, "If any of you object to completing the charts—just stand up, and I'll tell you what to do." He offered to accept anyone's resignation who was dissatisfied. Strange as it may seem, no one took him up on the proposition.

We were late in getting our checks, but it is just as well, as all our money (or over ½ of it) went across the street to the drug store. Boy, I'll bet the interns and residents are the main support of that store. But they are awfully good to us—send our watches in to be fixed, mail packages, sell us stamps, etc. It saves us many a trip downtown.

I do wish I might be looking around some for apartments, but I get tired pretty easily and have been trying to rest all I can. And I won't have much chance on OB. All I ask is not to be on night duty when you come—and gee, that won't be so long now, thank goodness.

Goodnight, sweetheart,
Alice

OMAHA
Wed. afternoon, May 31
4:40

My own sweetheart:

This room is about 100° hotter than the melting point of steel on these afternoons. The sun just beats in, and drawing the shades does not help very much.

Gee, the surgeon's temper went up 10 points with every hemorrhoid we got to the operating room this a.m. He let me do two of them—and again remarked that I should learn to tie knots better. But it's so much easier to tie them with string rather than suture.

Intravenous fluids galore—gee, I think I could do them in my sleep.

I am so anxious about your new service. I do hope you get some time off. Any arrangement must be better than the one that we have.

5:30

I wish those insurance salesmen would stay out. It seems that every football player becomes a salesman &, knowing my weakness for the game, they all come here. Again & again I tell them I have enough. $6,500 with a yearly premium of $108 is just plenty.

About the instructions, sweetheart, the diocese of Omaha does require them. I didn't know until I saw my priest that I do have to receive a dispensation for marriage from him—and that requires that he give you 6 short instructions. Since you are not here he suggested that they be given in N.O. I am sorry that I did not know about it sooner, but they did not require it in the diocese of Alexandria. So please, darling, would you do that for me? I am sorry that I cannot attend with you, and perhaps I can attend a few in July with you. But don't be afraid to ask anything, and I am sure the priest is better qualified to explain a lot of things than I am. But, darling, I know that we will not have any difficulties. Our roads may be different but the destination is the same.

And again I say, sweetheart, I will never ever try to force religion or anything else upon you. We will always be perfectly happy because we have practically everything in common—and I know that religion, in which we differ only in practice & some principles, will not mar it in the least.

I love you, sweetheart,

Joe

NEW ORLEANS

Fri. a.m., June 2

My dearest Joe—

I'll bet you never had a letter written to you at this time of night—or morning, I should say. Yes, 3:30 and all is well—finally. Five deliveries since 7—and now a toxemic patient, just delivered, to check blood pressure on every 30 minutes. I hope she calms down soon so I can get some rest, too.

It was terrible here for a while. All the babies were precipitating, but I slipped in on one and scrubbed before waiting for the nurses to call me, and I think I'll have to keep it up. At least I got to do one delivery correctly.

I slept pretty well today, better than I expected, but I assure you no one will have to tell me a bedtime story to get me to sleep this morning at 8. I brought my radio up here for amusement, but this darned old building has DC current and I expect it didn't do those radio tubes any good.

With so much time on my hands today, I became very ambitious. I made a trip to the record room and found, to my surprise, that I was only behind on 5 charts. Then I decided to do my good turn and write letters. So I wrote home and to Mary. Poor Mary, I've been owing her one for ever so long, but I surely had a lot of good news to tell her. Gee, I wish she might come down for our wedding. Wouldn't that be swell?

It's time to check the BP again—I'll see you later—

Oh, it is gradually coming down. Maybe I can get her out of the delivery room after awhile. I didn't understand the rationale of that infusion of 20% glucose on a hypertensive case right after delivery, but they say in these eclamptics, the blood pressure often falls very low. Gee, hers surely didn't.

Oh, it is nice and cool here—especially for me, since I just got a bath in amniotic fluid. I changed all the clothes I could up here decently, but still feel slightly damp. And I delivered my first baby with intact membranes, too. Gee, we promised the mother that boy would be a wonder! I expect she'll agree in more ways than one during the next few years.

The night supervisor just called us in for a snack—French toast and coffee. Gee, did it taste grand.

Dearest, it seems to me we are the most fortunate couple living. Yes, won't it be fun going home to our own little apartment and being together in everything. We'll have 2 years of separation to make up for before we even start on our full lifetime of happiness—and in less than a month, we can be together.

I love you, dearest one—
Alice

NEW ORLEANS
Sat. a.m., June 3
5:15

My beloved—

Oh, I was just awakened with "Her pains are pretty close together now." Well, they are, but she isn't fully dilated yet. And I was sleeping so well—Oh, well, here's a new patient to work up anyway.

7:10

Whew—a delivery, a false alarm, and now a patient has suddenly started bleeding. We're not allowed to touch a bleeding patient, and she was a pre-eclamptic anyway. I wonder if it could be a placenta previa. So far I've kept one ahead of the intern on day delivery. He had 3 yesterday and I had four last night. I'm really enjoying the service, and I think I'll soon get used to the night work. I got almost two hours of sleep last night.

We have one pitiful case here—a patient with a huge unusual hernia and a breech presentation. Her uterus seems thin-walled anyway, and she's been in labor for over 36 hours with no progress. The resident thinks she should have a section, but the visiting staff won't allow it. I surely think she should have one, but I guess they know what they are doing.

Darling, I understand about the instructions, but what do you mean that you have to have a dispensation for the marriage? I do hope I'm not interfering too much. I know, dearest, that you would never try to force anything on me. I know it and love you for it. I do wish we might have been of the same religion, but I think we shall be able to work out everything alright. Religion shouldn't be a point to cause separation between people in my opinion.

Boy, did I have a delicious steak—just rare enough to be juicy and good—with fresh buttered toast and orange juice. It was almost worth working at night for. It will be a habit very easy to acquire.

Gretchen is going home next week. Everyone is very pleased about her progress, and she is to go to work in October with the understanding that she has no night work. Is she happy!

I got a surprise yesterday—two dear letters from you. Gee, just think, 26 more days and I can receive my letters in person. Darling, I can hardly wait for those days to pass.

All my love,
Alice

NEW ORLEANS
Mon. Night, June 5

My beloved—

Surprise—I am no longer an obstetrician. Yes, Miss O'Dell phoned me today to tell me I would take over Frances' ward—the same old 522, colored G.U. which I had just started on when I had to go home in December. Frances tried to get them to let me stay on in OB, but they informed her I was extra and I needed to finish my G.U. service anyway.

I don't mind so much. I got enough deliveries to feel in the swing again, and I'm glad to have the easy service, for Mother and I must finish our shopping and this way, best of all, I can be sure of having my nights free while you are here.

Rudy Vallee—the "Beer Barrel Polka"—and was it good! I'd like to see the sparkle in your eyes when you hear that. I can just see them dancing.

Then I went on an ambulance ride with Dr. Edward F. Kelly. You should have heard everyone warning me about riding with a Yankee (he's from Michigan), but I still maintain that Yankees—at least, certain of them—can't be bettered. In fact, one of them is the dearest person in the world to me. Oh, darling, I am so anxious for June 29th.

Alice

NEW ORLEANS
Tues. Night, June 6

My dearest one—

I had quite a surprise today. I walked in at 7 p.m.—and there was Mother. Gee, was I glad to see her! We'll have to go shopping tomorrow. I do hope we can get everything done quickly on account of one sick patient. As far as the rest of them go, I might as well not be there. They'll get along fine without me.

We celebrated by going out to dinner and a show. Mother bought me a few dresses, but I'm trying to get her to take them back. I want to save all my new things for my trousseau. Oh, darling, I want to wear them first for you.

I'm getting the idea that we may be getting ourselves into a spot, in a way. I've already heard hints that the residents were going to resent our newly made authority. This wrinkle may have its few bad points, but surely it will work out OK. I just thought I'd give you a hint before you come as it has been brought to my attention.

Oh, but darling, what do we care? We can lick the whole world together. I love you and am so proud of you and so happy in my dreams of the future.

Goodnight, my sweetheart,
Alice

NEW ORLEANS
Wed. Night, June 7

My dearest one—

Today has been one full of thrills—but every moment of it there was an aching loneliness in my heart for you. First the secretary of the Medical Dept. at LSU asked me to come to the office to sign an application. It is the application for our rating with Charity Hospital. Our title was that of Assistant Visiting Physician. After signing mine she told me I could sign yours, too, for you wouldn't be here by June 15th and she would sign it if I didn't. So, darling, you see I have started a bad habit already, forging your name. But it made me so happy and relieved to know for sure you had your contract. Gee, I was just a slight bit worried but now, why, I haven't a care in the world.

Then we went shopping and I had another thrill—I selected my wedding dress. I wish you could see it—but that is supposed to be bad luck. At any rate, when you do see it, I shall be so blissfully happy! Oh, it seems the time will never pass—22 more days before I can see you.

Gee, I haven't earned my 33 1/3¢ today. I worked 1½ hours and was through for the day. My darling, I am now in a state of continuous suspense. My longing increases by the minute.

All my love,
Alice

OMAHA

Thu. Night, June 8

8:40

My sweetest one:

Golly, what a vivid picture they are painting of a hospital on Bing's program. That business of being awakened at 5 in the a.m. is right—particularly at the Pest House.

My patients are leaving one by one—some of them walking—and admissions are cut down since interns will change soon. Got in what appeared like a red hot appendix, but it's an inflammation of the fallopian tubes, so there was no surgery.

Sweetheart, will you be satisfied with Frances Langford's version of "Harbor Lights"? It was like a dream to listen to that selection again—my heart has not slowed down yet. Also got Bing in "The One Rose," "Dancing Under the Stars," "Now It Can Be Told" and some others. Now we have to rig up a phonograph attachment to your radio so we could play them any time. Won't they sound nice in years to come—oh, darling, it will be wonderful. I'm going to take extra special care of those records.

Cedarblade is all happy too. He will be married the first week in July. This business of marriage is rather epidemic around here. But, darling, none can be as happy as we will be.

Goodnight, Sweetheart,

Joe

New Orleans

Fri. Night, June 9

My dearest one—

Mother left this morning. My, but I enjoyed her visit. And, believe it
or not, I worked all morning and 1½ hours this p.m.

Say, they asked me what size coat you wore—you know, the long
white coat. I supposed a 38 extra long, but I can change it if that
isn't right. Won't it be fun to wear them?

Well, darling, I started the instructions today. I looked up the
hospital chaplain. There are two priests here, Father Robert Miget
and Father James Thompson. I asked the operator to get in touch
with one of them and it was the former. He is very nice, and as he
plans to leave for a vacation June 19th, he will give the instructions
every day except Sunday. He will write to Father Nuedling and send
him my pledges. He said everything should work out alright if you
have your baptismal certificate. I feel rather dumb but I thought
you had yours. I truly enjoyed the talk. It held just one disappointment—the explanation that you wouldn't be allowed to attend my
church services. I'm wondering if I may go to Mass with you.

Darling, I do hope I shan't interfere with your religious life. I
shan't intend to—I do so want not to impede you at all. But my
dearest, I love you wholeheartedly.

Goodnight, sweetheart,

Alice

NEW ORLEANS

Sat. Night, June 10

My beloved—

Darling, I miss you so much tonight I can hardly bear it. Ah, these days are dragging by so slowly. The memories of all our lovely times together are like twinkling stars in a dark night, but the thought of the loveliness of being with you soon is as brilliant as the sun.

We have tastes in common with Father Thompson. The "Beer Barrel Polka" is also a favorite of his. By the way, I had two more instructions today. Father Miget says Alexandria is in the N.O. diocese so he can fix up everything for us with less trouble.

Those talks are certainly interesting. He gave me some good advice about how to get along with a person even though married. Of course, I know that he is right. Little unpleasant things are bound to pop up. But I truly can't imagine it with you. Darling, you are perfect and so wonderful to me. And I'm so anxious for you to meet everyone.

I shall be so proud for you to meet Father Miget.

Then he will understand why I agree so perfectly with the perception that marriage is one and indissoluble—and means infinite trust and confidence.

Oh, dearest, my faith in you is truly infinite.

I love you,

Alice

OMAHA

Thu. Night, June 15

My adorable darling:

The chips are just flying in the card room. It seems someone brought up a new game called "7 Up." Almost as bad as "Cut Throat."

Gradually this service is cutting down, and I hope by the last week of June there will be no new cases. It seems I'll have to carry both surgery services for a few days before I leave. The histories will be brief and lab work nil. Only one intern is arriving early—which complicates things as far as my getting off early—but I still insisted I must be in N.O. June 29th.

Two other fellows are going down with me. We plan to leave the a.m. of the 27th and get to N.O. sometime about noon of the 29th. I'd like to stop at Alex to see your folks for a few hours on the way down. And then I have to make the definite time arrangement with Father Nuedling for the wedding. Gee, I'll be so glad to see your parents. They have always been so very, very nice to me. I'll never forget Christmas there. That fishing trip with your father. I enjoyed ward rounds with him and especially the stories of southern Indiana. I hope we can see a lot of them next year and always.

Do you realize, sweetheart—that one year ago tonight we were together at a show in New Iberia? And remember the dances we had at that little night club later? I'll bet everyone there saw that lovelight in our eyes. But, best of all, darling, was a year ago last night—the moon as we sat in Nola listening to Kay Kyser, and then that kiss. Sweetheart, my heart still pounds when I think of that.

Then there were those moments of ideal happiness we spent together traveling through all Southern Louisiana, then the nights in N.O. and all of your friends. Darling, every minute that we spend together will be a repetition of these heavenly moments of perfect bliss.

Only 14 more days. I wish time had the speed of light until then. After that, dearest, it can stop.

Goodnight, Sweetheart,

Joe

My beloved sweetheart—

I had a very nice letter from your Mother. Yes, it won't be long until she can call me her daughter. How happy that shall make me. I certainly am going to have the best in-laws anyone could have. You bet we are lucky to have the fathers and mothers that we have.

Gee, this is the fourth letter I've written tonight—I'm quite proud of myself. It always seemed to be a job to write letters until I started writing to you. Now it is the day's most pleasant occupation, but I shall be very glad to trade it for a real visit with you in person before long.

Oh, did you just hear Kay Kyser sing "Roll out the barrel?" Gee, I like that song. I wonder why. May I dance it with you sometime, pretty please?

Oh, darling, we are having such lovely cool starlight nights—and soon the moon will be full. The perfect setting for that perfect time when my sweetheart will be here. Oh, won't that lake be lovely? I'm counting on you finding a more private space than I did, though.

Goodnight, sweetheart,
Alice

NEW ORLEANS
Thurs. Nite, June 22

My dearest one—

Today has been another long, boring one. I had only one delivery in my 8 hours on duty. They had two ready for section—as soon as the visiting doctor could get to the hospital. One was a placenta previa, partial—about 80%. She had been bleeding quite profusely today, more than usual they say. The other was a toxemic patient with a generally contracted pelvis. I saw the resident 2 hours later and the visiting physician hadn't come yet.

I start working from 4 p.m. to midnight tomorrow, but it will be only 5 days. Then I shall have the ward during the daytime. Gee, hope I can get all those urines run by 6 p.m. anyway.

I stopped by the landladies' to tell them to expect you Thurs. and me Fri. nite. Their rooms are full now but they hope some of their roomers will leave within the week. If they don't, they will fix us up anyway. Bernes and Babe, her roommate, live just across the street so we may double up with them if necessary. In fact, you have been invited to sleep on the daybed in their front room. I declined for you but said I might take it—don't you wish I would keep out of your business?

Bernes is starting on her vacation tomorrow night, but she is going to save two days for our wedding. I'm so glad she can be there for it.

Did you notice the latest development of La. politics? Gov. Richard Leche is to resign because of ill health—and he is the youngest governor we have ever had. Rumors are flying thick and fast. Several things have been coming to light—WPA men building barns, etc., on the governor's private property, LSU trucks found furnishing LSU materials for private construction, etc. And if they start investigating where the money for the new hospital has gone, there might be several resignations because of ill health.

Of course, all the above is only rumor, and we're very sorry Gov. Leche is ill, etc., etc., etc.

Darling, I do hope you like it down here in spite of above. This much I assure you—I love you dearly—

Alice

CLARKSON

Mon. night, June 26

My adorable one:

It does feel good to be home again. It seems the only time I did spend here this year was while I was ill.

Father and Mother came for me today & we came home this evening. Gee, the car works swell. She has a constant desire to go south.

We plan to visit Adela and Louis tomorrow. Had some new pictures of Dennis taken and gee, but he is big. I bet I don't even recognize him tomorrow.

It did feel funny to leave the hospital—but when I thought of what ideal happiness is in store for us, that is all that mattered.

Am trying to plan a route for my trip now—undoubtedly Kansas City and Ft. Smith.

We have started to make a list for invitations—not over 10.

Had a nice visit with Grandmother tonight. She is a dear old soul—is getting cataracts now. She asks about you.

The folks send you their regards and love and are very anxious for the wedding. It will be 3 weeks from tomorrow.

Again, I cannot even start to tell you how I love you. I'll do my best to tell you the 30th.

I'll probably not write anymore—and I'm counting the hours until I hold you in my arms again.

Goodnight, Sweetheart,

Joe

EPILOGUE

Alexandria, New Orleans & Shreveport

"I agree so perfectly with the perception that marriage is one and indissoluble—and means infinite trust and confidence. Oh, dearest, my faith in you is truly infinite."

~Alice to Joe, June 10, 1939

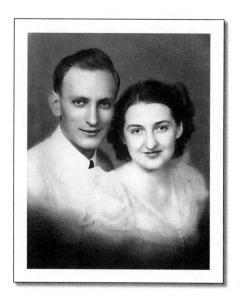

TUESDAY MORNING VOWS, a wedding breakfast, a stop at the photo studio—and Alice Baker and Joe Holoubek were off to begin their long-awaited life as not two but one.

July 18, 1939, was the beginning of the time Joe so clearly foresaw in his letters—"the heavenly days and years to come when we will be inseparable, professionally & socially."

But their day of bliss was not without a last-minute attack of nerves.

"Father Nuedling," Joe recalled later, "had early signs of Parkinson's, and my hands shook as badly as his."

The day was still vivid in his memory decades afterward.

"I feared for days that I would stutter when I said, 'I do.' When the time came, I flushed. My mouth opened but I could not speak. Alice looked at me, squeezed my hand, moved a little toward me, and the words 'I do' came out. The other words, with the rings, came a little easier. And soon it was over. We were man and wife. Then the kiss— and what a relief. I did it with Alice's help."

That set the tone for the rest of their lives—a couple who could accomplish far more together than they could separately. They would team in research, medical education, patient care, and personal causes, living up to the ideals each had recognized in the other the summer they met. They found great joy in their togetherness. One worry, however, could never quite be buried—that the lesion Alice had developed as an intern would indeed prove to be tuberculosis.

JOE'S FIRST TWO WEEKS in New Orleans set the pattern for their professional partnership. "Dr. Hull gave us our orders," he wrote later in one of several memoirs. "Hospital rounds every morning. Clinic every day. Tuesday and Thursday, pneumothorax in the TB hospital—injecting air into the cavity between the lung and the chest wall to collapse the lung and let it heal. In the fall, we would teach physical examination, physical diagnosis, and laboratory techniques. Then we were to do some research too. Alice and I had a good-sized office with laboratory facilities."

He and Alice barely had time to find an apartment, so involved were they with work and clinical care. "My first assignment was colored female. It was held in a building across Tulane Avenue. I went on the ward and saw malaria, beriberi, and all sorts of illnesses, some I had never before seen. I needed Alice by my side. At noon we ate at Joe's drug store across the street. I told her that I had to learn fast—and she helped me.

"Everyone was nice to me and treated me like I was one of them—I believe that they had so much respect for Alice. I continued to see patients with new diseases almost daily and kept asking Alice about them. She taught me well."

The entire hospital was moved into the new Charity during the two weeks Joe and Alice were married and on their honeymoon trip to Nebraska. It was several more weeks before they learned their way around the mammoth new hospital. Soon thereafter they plunged into their first research project—a study of tuberculosis in LSU medical students.

"We did TB tests on the students and took X-rays of the chest. We found 61 percent of the freshmen had been exposed to TB, 84 percent of the sophomores, 96 percent of the juniors, and 98 percent of the seniors. We found three students with active TB and six with arrested TB. The three students were started on pneumothorax during the Christmas vacation and did not miss school. After this research, LSU started a student health program.

"The research was first published in *The Tiger,* the medical school newspaper, and later in the *American Journal of Tuberculosis*. It was great to see an article published by Alice E. Baker M.D. and Joe E. Holoubek M.D."

Alice soon added her husband's name to hers professionally as well as socially, Joe recalled. "But not many could pronounce Holoubek so they called me Dr. Joe Baker."

Dr. Hull started the couple on another project—reviewing all autopsies between 1935 and 1939, determining which deaths were due to cardiac disease, then studying each case. They spent weeks in the pathology library. "We went over 10,000 autopsies and found 1,000 had died from heart disease. All of these were classified, and we eventually had four articles published in the American Heart Journal. Conditions that were then common—syphilitic heart disease, aortic aneurysm, and subacute bacterial endocarditis—have since disappeared due to antibiotics."

IN JUNE 1941, Joe's reserve unit in Nebraska activated. He was assigned to LaGarde Army Hospital, a 1,000-bed hospital being built on the lakefront in New Orleans. Only two weeks after he reported for duty, however, his worst fear was realized. Alice's TB was back.

A routine chest plate showed her lesion had spread.

"Bed rest *stat*," Joe jotted tersely in his journal. "We were a couple of depressed kids. Took a long last ride down Canal Street."

The next day, after giving Alice a complete physical, Dr. Hull recommended a year's leave of absence from her work. He did not push what other doctors suggested—an aggressive round of pneumothorax treatment. He favored instead a conservative watch-and-wait regimen.

Even so, Joe spent the day "walking around in circles." He could not help but remember the shock he felt in December 1938 upon first learning of Alice's lesion. "I had been a lot more worried than I let on," Joe recalled. "I had never seen a TB patient get well, and I feared she would become an invalid like all of the patients that I had seen in the Douglas County TB Hospital—thin, emaciated, and literally helpless.

"But I did not see my Alice as a lifelong tubercular, or consumptive, as we called it. I knew that the Lord had some other plan for her."

Once again, he hoped and prayed for the best. "If she had to stay in bed, so be it. I would support her."

Rest and inactivity proved again to be all that was needed, and by Christmas 1941, Alice was up and about. Several months later Alice went back to work part time, to help relieve a severe staff shortage at LSU. After Pearl Harbor, several members of the clinical and teaching staff of LSU medical school had taken military leave. Others formed the 64th General Hospital unit, which activated in

July 1942. Meanwhile, students were taking an accelerated schedule of courses to graduate early and accept commissions in the Army, Navy, or public health service.

At LaGarde, one medical officer after another was sent overseas, but hypertension kept Joe stateside throughout the war. Eventually his classification was changed to "limited duty," but he continued his work running the officers' ward and women's ward at the hospital.

Alice left work again—this time to prepare for their first child, a daughter, born in April 1943. While some doctors, all too aware of the risks to mothers with TB, advised terminating the pregnancy altogether, she and Joe entrusted her care to Dr. Hull. His calm was reassuring.

The danger, he argued, wasn't the pregnancy itself. It was exhaustion after the child was born. In fact, the pressure on the abdominal wall of carrying a baby offered a relief similar to collapsing the lung. At Hull's direction, the new parents arranged for help with child care so Alice could stay in bed for one month after their daughter was born and rest often thereafter.

Two years later, however, when Alice again became pregnant, she developed cavities in her right lung. Dr. Hull collapsed the lung and ordered twice-weekly pneumothorax treatments. She gave birth to their second child, a son, in February 1945.

Alice and Joe had planned to return to LSU School of Medicine to teach once the war ended. By late 1945, however, the school was on the verge of closure. High-handed politics and a new dean prompted mass resignations. Dr. Hull, then chairman of the Department of Medicine, was one of the last holdouts on the board.

Joe couldn't wait for matters to resolve themselves. He needed a job. He had two children and a wife with TB. His colonel at LaGarde, a Shreveport physician, offered him a position in private practice at $350 a month.

"That sounded good and we took it," he recalled later. They found a new three-bedroom house in Shreveport for $7,500.

"When I told Dr. Hull that we were going to Shreveport, he was glad. He had interned there and set up practice nearby. He said, 'They need a medical school in Shreveport.'"

Joe would never forget that remark.

ALICE WAS THE THIRD woman doctor to join the Shreveport Medical Society. She worked part time at Gilmer Chest Hospital, and she founded the Gabriel Group, a series of lectures for first-time mothers. Joe began to develop a following as a consulting cardiologist, internist, and diagnostician.

The two of them became involved in a new Catholic church a block from their home. The young pastor, the Rev. Joseph Gremillion, encouraged parishioners to bring the teachings of Christ into their work lives, brought young professionals together to "rub minds," and fostered an interest in social justice. "Father Joe" became the couple's close friend and spiritual director, and Alice converted to Catholicism in 1950.

A second son was born in 1948 and a second daughter in 1951. Then suddenly—full-blown TB. An X-ray showed a diffuse infiltration throughout Alice's right lung. "It was almost like galloping tuberculosis," Joe wrote years later. There were no antibiotic treatments as yet.

Dr. Hull came up and ordered total bed rest. Within one week, all of the arrangements were made—a Hungarian refugee would take care of the children. The nuns at the church prayed for Alice's recovery, and Gremillion asked for more prayers throughout the parish.

"We called the children together," Joe recalled, "and told them their mother needed at least six months in bed. This was a major blow. And we prayed."

Dr. Peachy Gilmer, the TB specialist, ordered another X-ray to measure how much the disease had spread in one week. He developed it and came back to take another picture. Then he brought out the old pictures and the new ones to show the Drs. Holoubek.

"The X-ray showed old calcified areas in the chest," Joe recalled. "This is the type of healing that the body does over a period of years in tuberculosis. The lesions of the TB are surrounded by fibrous tissue, which calcifies in time, and anyone looking at the picture can see the calcifications and call it old, healed TB. But this takes years to develop. Yet here she went from diffuse infiltration to old healed calcified tuberculosis in one week. That is medically impossible.

"Dr. Hull saw the pictures and said, 'Thank the Lord.' And thank Him we did. There is no doubt in my mind that this was a direct act of God."

> *"There is still much to be done in the field of medicine, and let us do our share—not for private and personal gain, but for the benefit of the profession and the multitude."*
> ~ Joe to Alice, November 12, 1937

> *"I hope I can someday be worthy of being called a 'real doctor' . . . which to me is the ultimate of human goodness, kindness, and helpfulness."*
> ~ Alice to Joe, November 29, 1937

WITH THEIR GREATEST WORRY behind them, Alice and Joe flourished personally and professionally. Working with several local doctors, they continued to do clinical research and publish their findings in medical and scientific journals. And once the children were in school, Alice joined Joe in private practice in internal medicine. Before long the firm of Holoubek & Holoubek became known as simply "Dr. Alice and Dr. Joe"—a term of both respect and endearment.

Patients understood that there was something more than diagnostics involved when they met with these physicians. As a Baptist preacher once told his family, "I learned more about Christianity from my doctor than anyone else."

In the early 1950s, the Holoubeks met Dr. Jean C. Brierre, who held medical degrees from the University of Haiti and McGill University in Montreal but was not allowed staffing privileges at Shreveport hospitals. "Racism was at its apogee," Brierre recalled later. "However, some men—Christian—were strong enough to take a stand and practice man's humanity to man." He and Joe, who shared an admiration for Louis Pasteur, became friends and confidants. They worked toward integrating hospital staffs and the Shreveport Medical Society.

Joe and Alice and friends also supported the founding of a local Friendship House, an interracial crusade to promote social justice. Father Gremillion was chaplain. Three staff members moved into a black neighborhood and presented weekly public forums on housing, voting rights, and other issues. After threats and intimidation and under pressure from the police, Friendship House closed about 18 months later. Gremillion later served Pope Paul VI as secretary of the Pontifical Commission on Justice and Peace.

Alice and Joe undertook several joint projects. They began a decades-long study of death by crucifixion, inspired by Dr. Pierre Barbet's groundbreaking work *A Doctor at Calvary* and by studies of the Shroud of Turin. This launched a series of talks on the physical sufferings of Christ throughout the region, across the nation, and in the Holy Land.

They developed interfaith marriage preparation programs for engaged couples that covered sexuality and health as well as legal, spiritual, and psychological issues.

They pioneered a preventive health program for priests, nuns, and other members of the clergy. Joe and Alice presented papers on the subject to the IX International Congress of Catholic Physicians in Munich and the Congregation of Religious and Clergy at the Vatican.

They also opened their home to a Catholic discussion group on matters of theology and morality. It met twice-monthly for nearly thirty years. Wilfred Guerin Ph.D., professor of English and future vice chancellor of LSU-Shreveport, was among the regular attendees. "The Monday gatherings provided for an intellectual exchange, for adult religious education, even for spiritual formation. . . . It was stimulating, it was a bonding, and it reflected love."

Joe took the more public role in the outside world, leading the National Federation of Catholic Physicians Guilds, the Louisiana Heart Association, and the Tri-State Medical Society. Alice became a role model for many local young women in balancing family, profession, and civic involvement. Bishop William Friend of the Diocese of Shreveport was among those impressed by Dr. Alice's quiet dedication. "In her dealings with the poor and the needy," he told the Shreveport *Times* years later, "Dr. Holoubek acted in such a way that she always brought respect to the poor and recognized their dignity."

All along, Joe and Alice pondered the parting words of their mentor, Dr. Edgar Hull, when they left New Orleans in 1945. His words inspired them to lead a drive for medical education in Shreveport.

Joe chaired the medical school development committee of the Shreveport Medical Society in the 1960s. Members mounted an intensive effort to secure state funding for the school, over the opposition of many people of influence. Without any paid lobbyists, they obtained the $10 million to start LSU School of Medicine in Shreveport by unanimous vote in Louisiana's House of Representatives and only one negative vote in the Senate. Dr. Hull was named the first dean—and the medical school quickly became the driving force of a regional health-care industry.

Decades later, John C. McDonald M.D., chancellor of LSU Health Sciences Center Shreveport, paid tribute to Joe's leadership. "Dr. Holoubek is a giant figure in the history of the LSU School of Medicine in Shreveport. He had a vision for a new medical school in Shreveport and worked tirelessly to make that vision reality."

"Darling, every breath is a prayer that we may find our happiness together. Goodnight, dearest sweetheart—"
~ Alice to Joe, April 23, 1939

DR. ALICE AND DR. JOE never stopped counting their blessings, starting with her health, their children and grandchildren, and their ever-fresh love for one another. After retirement, they pursued their interest in religion, taking more than forty courses in the Scriptures, theology, Biblical history, and early Christianity. And they kept presenting talks on the Passion of Christ.

They marked their fortieth anniversary, their fiftieth, their sixtieth. The couple who married seven months after a TB diagnosis enjoyed longer lives than they could ever have imagined. But they had to deal with the same kind of illnesses they once treated in aging patients—frailty and loss of memory. When they could no longer dance to "Harbor Lights" or any other of their favorite tunes, they enjoyed pulling out the letters of their courtship and reading them to each other.

In 1993, after one long hospitalization, Joe turned to writing fiction. Close to death at one point, he had dreamed he was in Nazareth when Jesus was expelled from the synagogue—a scene recounted in the gospel of St. Luke—but had not defended him. Guilt lingered until he took pen to paper, expressing what was in his heart as he once had to the girl from Louisiana. Over the next ten years, he drew from the deep wells of his faith, his knowledge, and his love for Alice, producing the award-winning *Letters to Luke: From His Fellow Physician Joseph of Capernaum.* The story of a man of science who becomes a man of faith, it is told through letters written by a first century physician. "I didn't know how to write fiction," Joe said later, "but I knew how to write letters."

C. Everett Koop, former U.S. surgeon general, pronounced the Bible-based novel "a unique way to present the gospel, the life of Luke, a smattering of medical history, and a love story."

The primary female character is Elisa of Capernaum, a brave and brilliant young woman trained in the healing arts. *Letters to Luke* was published in 2004, seven months before the death of his beloved Alice.

Joe never lost his fascination with the girl from Louisiana.

APPENDIX

Timeline

July	1937	Joe Holoubek of Nebraska and Alice Baker of Louisiana meet during summer fellowship program in pathology, Mayo Clinic, Rochester
September	1937	Senior years of medical school begin, Omaha and New Orleans
April	1938	Joe finishes thesis
May/June	1938	Joe and Alice graduate from medical school
June 14–22	1938	Joe visits Louisiana with parents, gives Alice his fraternity pin
July 1	1938	Internships begin, Omaha and New Orleans
Sept. 13–17	1938	Alice visits Omaha and Clarkson; Joe and Alice travel to Rochester
November	1938	Joe is hospitalized briefly
Dec. 7	1938	Alice is sent home on bed rest
Dec. 24–31	1938	Joe visits Alexandria, gives Alice a ring
January	1939	Joe is sent to the isolation hospital in Omaha
February	1939	Joe resumes internship
March	1939	Joe is again hospitalized briefly
April 1	1939	Alice resumes internship
May	1939	Alice and Joe accept fellowship offer
July 1	1939	Alice and Joe begin fellowship
July 18	1939	Alice and Joe marry

Family and Friends

Joe Edward Holoubek was the son of Marie Kucera and Joseph Holoubek and brother to Adela Holoubek Sedlak. Other relatives named in the letters are brother-in-law Louis Sedlak and nephew Dennis Sedlak. Adolf "A.C." Cimfel, also a medical student from Clarkson, was like a member of the family. Joe had pet names for family vehicles—Nancy, Nellie, Nola, and Noma—and for his camera, Argus.

Alice Elizabeth Baker is the daughter of Effie Maud Wiseman and Erasmus Shanks Baker M.D. and sister to Polly Baker Miller and Ray Baker M.D. Other relatives named in the letters are aunt Mary Baker, uncle Charlie Baker, and sister-in-law Marie Baker. Clotile Sandres kept house for the Bakers. Their family car was dubbed Happy.

Dr. John and Bea Tyson, parents of infant John Charles, were friends of the family; Dr. Tyson was a staff physician at U.S. Veterans Hospital in Pineville, Louisiana.

Friends in New Orleans included Bernes Larson, a dietitian at Hotel Dieu Hospital, and radiology resident Dorothy ("Dot") Mattingly, sister of a Charity Hospital surgeon. In Rochester, Alice roomed with former Louisiana resident Mary Lomasney; their fathers had worked together at Veterans Hospital.

Medical Professionals

(Physicians, professors, and instructors named in the letters)

NEBRASKA

University of Nebraska College of Medicine, University of Nebraska Hospital, Creighton University School of Medicine, Nebraska Methodist Hospital, and private practice, all in Omaha

Baker, Dr. Charles	Pathologist, Nebraska Methodist Hospital
Bean, Dr. Francis	Assistant superintendent, University Hospital
Clark, Dr. Mildred Johnson	Obstetrics-gynecology, University Hospital
Cloyd, Dr. Augustus David	Instructor, medicine, UN
Eggers, Dr. Harold	Professor, pathology and bacteriology, UN
Hall, Dr. Lynn T.	Assistant professor, medicine, UN
Heine, Dr. Lyman	ENT, University Hospital
Henske, Dr. J.A.	Pediatrics, University Hospital
Hicken, Dr. N. Frederick	Surgery, University Hospital
Judd, Dr. John Hewitt	Instructor, otolaryngology, UN
Keegan, Dr. J.J.	Professor, surgery, UN
Kennedy, Dr. Charles Rex	Professor, surgery, UN
Kirk, Dr. E.J.	Associate professor, medicine, UN
Luikart, Dr. Ralph	Associate professor, obstetrics, Creighton
Mason, Dr. Claude	Assistant professor, medicine, UN
McCarthy, Dr. Joseph D.	Assistant professor, medicine, UN
McLaughlin, Dr. Charles	Assistant professor, surgery, UN
Nelson, Dr. Floyd C.	Family physician, Omaha
Nillson, Dr. John R.	Surgery, University Hospital
Poynter, Dr. Chas. Wm. McCorkle	Dean, UN College of Medicine, 1930–1946
Pratt, Dr. George	Associate professor, medicine, UN
Prichard, Dr. George	Instructor, medicine, UN
Sage, Dr. Earl Cuddington	Director, Department of OB-Gyn, UN
Shearer, Dr. William L.	Director, Department of Oral & Facial Surgery, UN
Stastny, Dr. Olga F. Sadilek	Instructor, OB-Gyn, UN
	Private practice, Omaha
	Croix de Guerre and other international

	medals for humanitarian work during and after World War I
Sucha, Dr. W.L.	Director, Department of Orthopedic Surgery, Creighton University team physician
Tomlinson, Dr. C. C.	Director, Department of Dermatology and Syphilology, UN

Students, interns, and residents, University of Nebraska College of Medicine and University of Nebraska Hospital, 1937–1939

Cedarblade, Dr. Vincent Gustave	
Cerv, Ernie *	
Cimfel, Dr. Adolf "A.C."*	
Dunn, Dr. Arthur	Resident, medicine
Drummond, Dr. Dave	Resident, pathology
Krausnick, Dr. Keith*	
McVay, Dr. Clark L.	Resident, obstetrics
Modlin, Dr. Herbert	
Richards, Dr. Francis	Resident, OB-Gyn
Ross, Dr. Donald	
Schmela, Dr. W.W.	Resident, radiology

*Nu Sigma Nu medical fraternity

LOUISIANA

Charity Hospital, LSU School of Medicine, Tulane University School of Medicine, and private practice in New Orleans; U.S. Veterans Hospital in Pineville; and Baptist Hospital in Alexandria

Allen, Dr. Charles	Instructor, medicine, LSU
Ashman, Dr. Richard	Director, Department of Physiology, LSU
Barker, Dr. Hiram O.	Superintendent, Baptist Hospital, Alexandria
Bauer, Dr. Julius	Instructor, medicine, LSU
Bayley, Dr. Robert	Assistant professor, medicine, LSU
Bel, Dr. George S.	Director, Charity Hospital Director, Department of Medicine, LSU
Brewster, Dr. H.F.	Clinical assistant professor, ophthalmology, LSU
Burns, Dr. Beryl Iles	Director, Department of Anatomy, LSU Dean, LSU School of Medicine, 1939–1945

Carter, Dr. Phillips John	Clinical professor, OB-Gyn, LSU
Casey, Dr. Albert	Assistant professor, pathology and bacteriology, LSU
Castellani M.D., Sir Aldo	Visiting professor, tropical medicine, LSU
Crawford, Dr. Rena	Clinical instructor, pediatrics, LSU
Dees-Mattingly, Dr. Marie Byrd	Associate professor, anatomy, Tulane
D'Anna, Dr. J.A.	Clinical professor, surgery, LSU
D'Aunoy, Dr. Joseph Rigney	Dean, LSU School of Medicine, 1937–1939
Echols, Dr. Dean Holland	Instructor, surgery, Tulane
Fuchs, Dr. Val Henry	Clinical professor, otolaryngology, LSU Director, postgraduate program
Goldsmith, Dr. Grace	Professor, medicine, Tulane
Granger, Dr. Amédée	Professor, radiology, LSU
Howles, Dr. James Kirby	Professor, dermatology and syphilology, LSU
Hull, Dr. Edgar	Professor (later department director), medicine, LSU Mentor of Alice Baker and Joe Holoubek
Jones, Dr. Will O'Daniel	Staff physician, Veterans Hospital, Pineville
Lowe, Dr. Robert Chester	Instructor, medicine, LSU
Maes, Dr. Urban	Director, Department of Surgery, LSU
Mattingly, Dr. Charles Walter	Senior visiting surgeon, Charity Hospital
Nix, Dr. James Thomas	Clinical professor, surgery, LSU
Schattenberg, Dr. Herbert John	Associate professor, pathology, Tulane
Schenken, Dr. John Rudolph	Director, Department of Pathology and Bacteriology, LSU
Weilbaecher, Dr. Joseph Oswald	Clinical assistant professor, medicine, LSU

Interns and residents, Charity Hospital, 1937–1939

Albritton, Dr. A. Stirling	
Bishop, Dr. Clarence	
Dupuy, Dr. Homer	
Evans, Dr. Frances E.	
Fader, Dr. David E.	Resident, medicine
Huff, Dr. W. Cloyce	
Irwin, Dr. James Barrett	Resident, radiology
Jernigan, Dr. Henry C.	

Kelly, Dr. Edward F.
Kleinsasser, Dr. L.J.   Resident, surgery
Lockhart, Dr. Ellanor*
Mattingly, Dr. Dorothy*   Resident, radiology
Tisdale, Dr. Alice M. Correll*
Vitter, Dr. Gretchen M.*   Resident, pathology
*Alpha Epsilon Iota medical sorority

MINNESOTA
Mayo Clinic, associated with Mayo Foundation and University of Minnesota Graduate School of Medicine, all in Rochester

Adson, Dr. Alfred	Senior neuro-surgeon, Mayo Clinic
Allen, Dr. Edgar V.	Consultant and head of internal medicine section, Mayo Clinic
Balfour, Dr. Donald	Consulting surgeon, Mayo Clinic and associated hospitals Director, graduate medical education
Bannick, Dr. Edwin G.	Assistant professor, medicine, Mayo Clinic
Bargen, Dr. J. Arnold	Associate professor, medicine, Mayo Foundation and UM Graduate School
Broders, Dr. A.C.	Surgical pathologist, Mayo Clinic Professor, pathology, Mayo Foundation and UM Graduate School
Gray, Dr. H.K.	Associate professor, surgery, UM
Hench, Dr. Philip S.	Consultant and head of internal medicine section, Mayo Clinic
Hildebrand, Dr. Alice Grace	Mayo fellow, internal medicine; graduate of UN College of Medicine
MacCarty, Dr. William Carpenter	Professor, pathology, UM Director, summer fellowship program
Rutledge, Dr. D. Ivan	Mayo fellow, internal medicine; graduate of UN College of Medicine
Wilder, Dr. Russell	Professor, internal medicine, UM

Sources

Among the materials consulted to ensure accuracy:

Charity Hospital-New Orleans annual reports, 1937–1940
LSU School of Medicine-New Orleans registers, 1938–1942
City directories, 1935–1940
    Alexandria-Pineville, Louisiana
    New Orleans, Louisiana
    Omaha, Nebraska
    Rochester, Minnesota
Directory of physicians in the United States, American Medical Association,
    1942
Directory of medical specialists certified by American boards. Paul Titus M.D.,
    ed. New York. Published for the Advisory Board for Medical Specialties by
    Columbia University Press, 1939.

Alumni records:

Alpha Epsilon Iota (directory-journal, 1944)
Gumbo (LSU yearbook), 1935–1938
LSU School of Medicine, New Orleans
Nu Sigma Nu (Beta Epsilon chapter) bulletin, 1938–1939, and photo, 1936
Reinert-Alumni Library, Creighton University, Omaha
University of Nebraska Medical Center, Omaha
Tulane University Health Sciences Center, New Orleans

Other archives and historical records:

Catholic Diocese of Alexandria, Louisiana
Loyola University, New Orleans
Mayo Clinic Historical Archives, Rochester, Minnesota
Mayo Foundation History of Medicine Library, Rochester, Minnesota
McGoogan Library of Medicine, University of Nebraska Medical Center,
    Omaha
Olmsted County History Center, Rochester, Minnesota
Rudolph Matas Medical Library, Tulane Health Sciences Center, New Orleans
A Century of Caring: 1889–1989. St. Marys Hospital of Rochester, Minnesota,
    1988
A History of LSU School of Medicine in New Orleans, Russell C. Klein M.D. and
    Victoria Barreto Harkin. New Orleans: LSU Medical Alumni Association,
    2010.

Inter⟍   ⟍, St. Marys
Hⱷ⟍ⱷⱷ⟍⟍⟍, ⟍⟍⟍⟍⟍⟍⟍⟍, ⟍⟍⟍

Personal papers of Dr. and Mrs. E.S. Baker. Private collection of Holoubek family.

Diaries and journals of Dr. Joe E. Holoubek. Private collection of Holoubek family.

The following archives own copies of *The Holoubek-Baker Letters, 1937–1939, An Annotated Collection*, Martha H. Fitzgerald, ed., Shreveport, 2008:

McGoogan Library of Medicine, University Of Nebraska Medical Center, Omaha

Mayo Clinic Historical Archives, Rochester, Minnesota

Medical libraries at the LSU Health Sciences Centers in New Orleans and Shreveport, Louisiana

LSU Shreveport Archives—Noel Memorial Library, Shreveport

LSUS archives also holds an extensive compilation of Holoubek memoirs, publications, and personal papers: *Collection 637, Drs. Alice (1914–2005) and Joe (1915–2007) Holoubek Collection, 1929–2007.*